# READ

# WITHOUT

## GLASSES

### AT ANY AGE

ALSO BY ESTHER JOY VAN DER WERF:

Available in paperback and as e-book:

*Bates Method Nuggets, The Fundamentals of Natural Vision Improvement by William H. Bates, M.D.* A compilation of the best of Dr. Bates' writings; clear and practical advice covering all aspects of his method.

Available as e-books:

*Better Eyesight magazines.* The complete, unedited, and searchable collection of Dr. Bates' monthly magazines which were originally published from July 1919 to June 1930.

The Bates Method View of – a series of e-books on various vision challenges:

- *The Bates Method View of Cataracts*
- *The Bates Method View of Conical Cornea*
- *The Bates Method View of Floaters*
- *The Bates Method View of Glaucoma*
- *The Bates Method View of Nystagmus*
- *The Bates Method View of Presbyopia*
- *The Bates Method View of Retinitis Pigmentosa*

*Eye Education in Our Schools.* Detailed examples of how the Bates Method was used in schools and the results that were obtained.

All are available from www.visionsofjoy.org

# READ

# WITHOUT

# GLASSES

## AT ANY AGE

**The Natural Way to Near Vision Clarity**

**by Esther Joy van der Werf**

*Foreword by Ray Gottlieb, O.D., Ph.D.*

Published by Visions of Joy, Ojai, California

ISBN: 978-1-935894-08-7

First Edition – Color Special

Published by Visions of Joy, Ojai, California. www.visionsofjoy.org
Printed by America's Press, www.americaspress.com
Printed in the United States of America

Cover design by Rick and Lisa Monzon. monzonart.blogspot.com
Illustrations on pages 1, 37, 38, 45, 55, 65, 79 by Rick Monzon
Illustration on page 60 by Leideke Steur, www.leidekesteur.nl
Illustration on pages 7 by Tatiana Swope with Esther Joy van der Werf
Other illustrations by Esther Joy van der Werf

I dedicate this book to my niece

***Ingeborg van Vlimmeren***

7 May 1987 – 4 March 2009

with deep gratitude for
the Love and Light
she radiated.

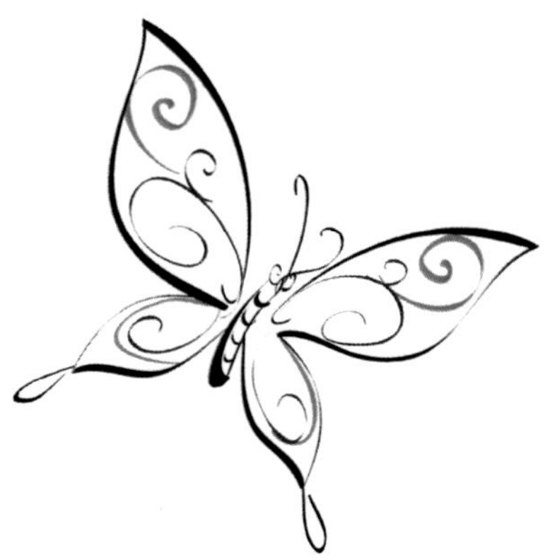

# Contents

# Acknowledgments

[12] The incredible work done by William H. Bates, M.D., and his wife Emily (Lierman) Bates forms the basis of this book. Dr. Bates was the pioneer in finding effective ways of improving eyesight naturally and Emily assisted his patients in successfully applying the doctor's knowledge for their vision improvement. I am so grateful that Dr. Bates and Emily published much of their research and case histories so their knowledge has remained available and continues to serve people world-wide.

I have deep gratitude for the Bates Method teachers who carried on Dr. Bates' work after his death. I feel blessed to have met dozens of colleagues at holistic vision conferences and consider many of them my friends. Their various insights into natural vision improvement helped shape me as a teacher.

Ray Gottlieb, O.D., Ph.D., broadened my scope on presbyopia beyond Dr. Bates' work. Ray also taught me about syntonics; the effects of color light therapy on vision. It is a real blessing to know Ray. I am grateful for his friendship and for his enthusiasm for this book. I feel so honored that he accepted my request to write the foreword!

I am also truly grateful for the many people who came to me seeking help for their presbyopic eyes, especially those who worked with the much smaller first version of this book and whose questions helped to evolve it. They too have been my teachers; I thank you all.

Sincere thanks go to my three editors who are also great friends: Sydney Sims, Ph.D., Lisa Harvey, O.D., and Moira Blaisdell. These amazing women caught a slew of spelling, grammatical, and punctuation errors. Lisa also provided valuable feedback which improved the content of this book.

Three dear friends deserve special mention: Charan van Tijn, Malcolm McKeand, and Bonnie Cornu. In the early phase of this book Charan's excellent questions caused me to enhance the clarity of various sections, while in the final phase Malcolm's listening ear helped me past some frustrating stumbling blocks. Bonnie has cheered me on ever since we met and has been my 'bestest' friend for more than a decade. I cannot express enough gratitude for the love, care, and support of these wonderful people in my life.

I am delighted that Rick and Lisa Monzon designed the cover and they provided the majority of the illustrations, so this book could go into print with a professional look!

Last but definitely not least, my heartfelt thanks to my loving parents, my dear sister, and my entire extended family, whose love and support enrich my life tremendously. I am so happy to be making this journey on earth with you. Ik hou van jullie. ♥

# Foreword

[12] Presbyopia (middle age sight) is the loss of near vision focus that forces billions of people to wear reading prescriptions around or after forty years old. In the conventional view, the inevitability of presbyopia is an unquestioned fact of aging that afflicts 100% of the population by age fifty. The assertion that presbyopia can be postponed, reversed or prevented through eye exercise is ridiculed by eye doctors and proponents are attacked as professionally irresponsible. I disagree. Vision training can postpone and reverse presbyopia and a growing number of eye professionals are starting to agree with me.

The conventional view of presbyopia is not an ironclad fact. Rather, it is a theory and theories are essentially guesses that are subject to change as new facts are discovered. William H. Bates, M.D., the father of natural methods of vision improvement, stated this in the preface to his 1920 book *Perfect Sight Without Glasses*:

> "In the science of ophthalmology, theories, often stated as facts, have served to obscure the truth and throttle investigation for more than a hundred years. The explanations of the phenomena for sight . . . have caused us to ignore or explain away a multitude of facts which otherwise would have led to the discovery of the truth about errors of refraction . . . "

Dr. Bates suggested an alternative model consisting of principles and practices for reversing rather than neutralizing (with glasses) a range of eye conditions. In my opinion, the most interesting of his writing was his personal experience in eliminating presbyopia in his own eyes.

I "cured" my mild (-1.25D) myopia in 1972 using Bates exercises and body therapy. It took me six months to learn how to voluntarily clear my distance seeing and another year until I could do this so quickly and automatically that I was essentially no longer nearsighted. Not only could I see better than 20/20 in each eye but objective tests showed that my eyes were normal (required zero diopters). In 1976, I invented a new presbyopia reduction approach to help a fifty-two year-old patient. It worked and not only reversed his presbyopia but also eliminated his farsightedness. I used it for years with my patients and in 2005 it was produced as a DVD called *The Read Without*

*Glasses Method.* These two natural practices have kept me glasses-free and clear sighted in each eye at near and far distance for more than three decades.

Presbyopia is the first obvious sign of aging. It forces us to confront the inevitable -- that we've passed our peak and are starting the slide towards old age. We don't want to see this and we don't want others to see it either. Many people seem to hate bifocals and resent the inconvenience of reading glasses, especially those who never needed glasses until presbyopia. This led to alternative approaches such as "monovision" contact lenses (where one eye was prescribed for seeing near details and the other for far). Invisible, no-line bifocal and then progressive or multifocal glasses and contacts were invented to hide presbyopia.

A growing number of new presbyopia treatments are just becoming available. Why now? Presbyopic baby-boomers are very interested in anti-aging and natural approaches in medicine. They are looking for alternatives. And once corporation leaders looking for new profit centers realized the potential of presbyopia treatments, the race was on.

In the last decade a number of bold surgical approaches has emerged: monovision Keratoplasty (reshaping the cornea using laser surgery or microwaves), IntraCor (a method of inserting bubbles in the cornea), Refractive Lens Exchange (removing the eye's natural lens to insert specialized variable artificial lenses by performing cataract surgeries on non-cataract patients), laser corneal surgery to resculpt the cornea as a multifocal lens, and surgery to insert or attach small lenses into or onto the cornea.

In addition two non-invasive light therapy approaches are being developed for presbyopia reduction. Transscleral Red Light Therapy shines infrared lasers on the white of the eye and Aculight applies narrow beams of colored light around the closed eye and onto other points on the head and body.

Self-health approaches such as yoga, jogging, diet, and teeth brushing are not quick fixes. They work only when done on a prolonged and regular basis. So too presbyopia reduction practices. Time and attention are the price you must pay. Just how much time each day depends on you, how fit and healthy you are, whether your body learns and adapts easily and in which phase of the process you are. In the initial phase you are learning how to practice without effort. It's very important to minimize fatigue, frustration and anxiety and to maximize motivation. If your initial expectations are too high and you work too hard, you'll lose motivation and quit. A teacher helps a lot at this stage.

Learning new skills takes time, especially if you are full of self-doubt about your learning or worry whether this pursuit actually can reduce presbyopia. In this case, you need to ease into the process, substitute curiosity for expectation, and practice for just a short time each day and maybe not every day. If you stay with it you will gain understanding, competence and trust and you will find yourself in the next phase where you enjoy the practice and are very motivated to dedicate large chunks of time to intense practice. You would practice all day, every day if you had the time, because it feels right and good. The result is that the process becomes automatic and you achieve success – your presbyopia is no longer a problem. In the final phase you work just enough to maintain your gains, more if you are ill or stressed and less if you are vital.

In my life, I have incorporated the Bates practices described herein. I do them all-day-long unconsciously even when I'm concentrating hard to navigate a difficult situation or learn a complex task. So it takes very little time out of my day. I don't practice my presbyopia exercise on a daily basis. I do it when I feel the need. Even now in my seventies I can go for weeks or months with no presbyopia symptoms and I don't need to practice. Other times I feel myself starting to strain to read small print and I need frequent practice for several days.

I'm pleased to see that Esther Joy van der Werf has written *Read Without Glasses at Any Age* now. Its publication brings a fresh look at Bates' work at a time when it's really needed. Her book gets straight to the point. It is free of fluff and true to Bates' approach and includes plenty of his original writing about his own and his patients' experiences of learning to see small print without artificial aids. Esther's little book takes just an hour or two to read but success comes by learning, doing and staying with the process until it becomes part of who you are, all day, every day for the rest of your life.

Ray Gottlieb, O.D., Ph.D.
July 2013

# Introduction

[21] Do you remember when you could easily read any size letters? It may have been recently or a long time ago. Back then you never even thought about your eyes while reading, now anything near your face is out of focus and you automatically grab your reading glasses as soon as text looks too small.

How will you feel if your clarity returns and the glasses are no longer needed? How much relief will you feel if you no longer need to keep track of where those darn glasses are?

Imagine easily reading menus by candlelight and impressing your friends by doing so with your own healthy eyes, free from crutches.

Or imagine no longer peering over glasses to see people across the room. Won't that be nice?!

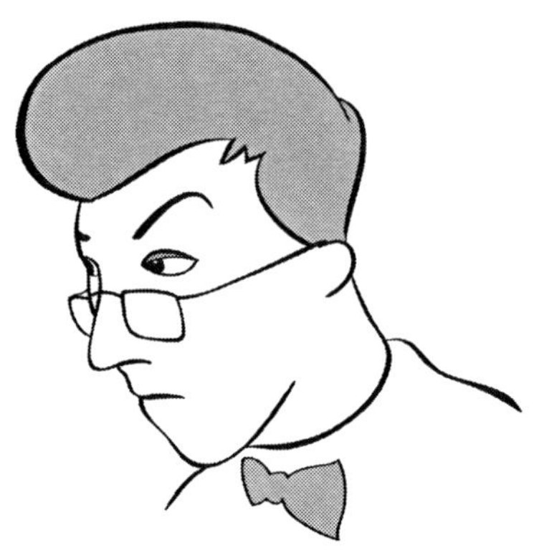

If these thoughts appeal to you, this book is for you!

Whether your age is 46-ish or 86+, and even if you are only six and just learning to read, this book can be a valuable tool to overcome your reading challenges.

The methods outlined in this book are simple, easy to learn and just as easy to apply. It does take some time and persistence, but the rewards are huge – a return to natural clear vision, healthier eyes, and easy, glasses-free reading.

Although this book is thorough and quite specific about parts of the Bates Method, it does not provide a complete overview of the entire method. My first book *Bates Method Nuggets* covered that already. My aim here is to provide you with the most effective tools for reading without glasses. No frills, no fancy exercises, no excess baggage. You get exactly the things you need to move from reading with glasses, to reading without them.

I believe this option to improve sight without glasses should be widely known and available. For individual help and guidance in the use of the Bates Method for general vision improvement, please contact your local teacher.[1]

I wish you all the best on your path to clarity!
Love & Light,

Esther Joy van der Werf
Ojai, California, July 2013

# How to Use this Book

[20] **You are invited…**
The large print in the early chapters of this book is an invitation for you to take off your glasses and start reading without them. You may be pleasantly surprised by how soon your eyes adjust to the gradually decreasing print size, yet if it seems too challenging at first, pages 21 to 23 have suggestions to bridge the visual gap.

[19] The following pages will serve as your guide through a ten-step process to reading without glasses. Each step will help you understand a part of the Bates Method and provides ways to apply it to your reading at a level suitable to your current ability. For that reason I highly recommend you take the steps in the order they are presented.

Allow plenty of time to become familiar with each step: an hour, a day, or longer. Anyone who has not yet used reading glasses can go through the steps faster than someone who has used readers for years. If you belong to the latter category, taking two or three steps per week is likely much better than two steps per day. Some steps will bring quick results, while others take time before you see their benefit.

[18] Everyone's needs are unique, so go through all the steps, and do the ones that work best for you most often. If you reach a plateau, come back to the other steps - you may find that your understanding of them changes and that you can put them to good use later.

**Different vision in each eye?**
Some people see better with one eye than the other. If this is the case for you, you will find specific advice on page 55 in step 4 to help balance your eyes.

## NOTES:

- Numbers in square brackets [18] denote the font size of paragraph(s) following it.
- Superscript numbers [21] refer to chapter notes at the end of the book.

## Have Your Arms Become Too Short?

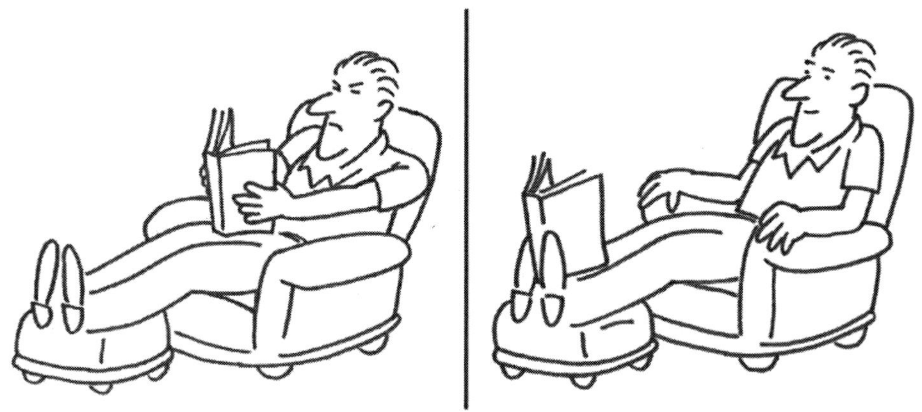

[25] Reading is usually the biggest challenge for farsighted people. You may feel that your arms are becoming too short as you have to hold print further and further away to see it clearly, or you need good light and larger print to read without glasses.

You may find yourself squinting much more to read, while reading for any length of time likely causes you to feel sleepy.

[24] Tilting your head back probably improves near vision clarity but strains your neck. Perhaps your only problem so far is that your eyes are slow to focus when shifting from far to near vision or back.[2] If you let any of these symptoms continue, chances are you will soon buy your first reading glasses.

Possibly you already own several pairs of reading glasses and your memory of the clear eyesight you used to enjoy has faded. What happened? How do your eyes focus and why might they fail? These are legitimate questions for which scientists have no clear answer yet. I will give you a brief overview of my understanding of current theories.

The ability of the eye to focus at different distances, also called the process of accommodation, is a reflex[3] with a variety of components. It begins with a mental shift in attention, for example: from a distant object to a near one. What follows that mental shift to a nearer object is generally believed to be:

The eyes converge (both eyes turn toward the nose to point at the nearer object); the cones (the retina's light-receptor cells that have the ability to see clearly) register blur and trigger a need to re-focus;[4] the pupils constrict (miosis; a reduction in pupil diameter, which is more common in adults); the ciliary body in each eye moves slightly forward as the ciliary muscles tense, which reduces tension on the zonules that hold the lens in place, which in turn allows the lens to become more rounded so the image of the near object focuses on the retina in the back of each eye.

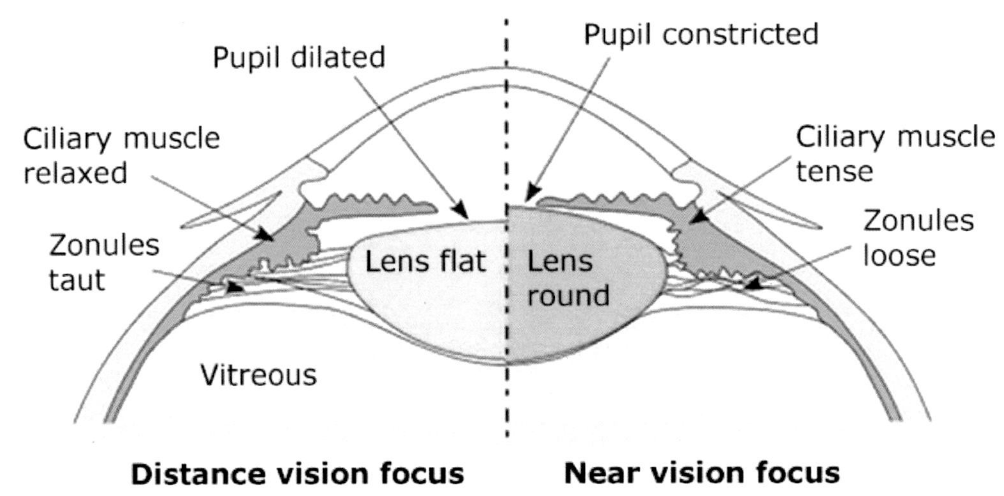


Interference in any part of this process can result in blurry vision at the near point.

[23] Various elements may play a role when focus fails at close range:

- the lens grows and hardens[2,5,6]
- the ciliary muscle may atrophy or become chronically tense[5,7-11]
- the zonules lose elasticity[12,13]
- the ciliary body's forward shift decreases[10]
- the pupil fails to contract sufficiently

To what extent each of these factors is involved remains under debate. Besides the above possible contributory causes, the influence of rest versus stress, a healthy or junk-food diet, general fitness or lack thereof and the amount of time glasses are used, are generally left out of the equation.

Presbyopia is a Latin word of Greek origin that literally means ‘old man eyes.’ It is the name given to the reduced ability of the eyes to focus at the near point as you age.

The chart on the next page shows the correlation between your focusing power (accommodative range of your eyes, measured in diopters) and the distance from your eyes (in centimeters) beyond which you can see clearly. You will notice that, as amplitude drops, the point of near vision clarity moves further out.

# Accommodative Amplitude Chart

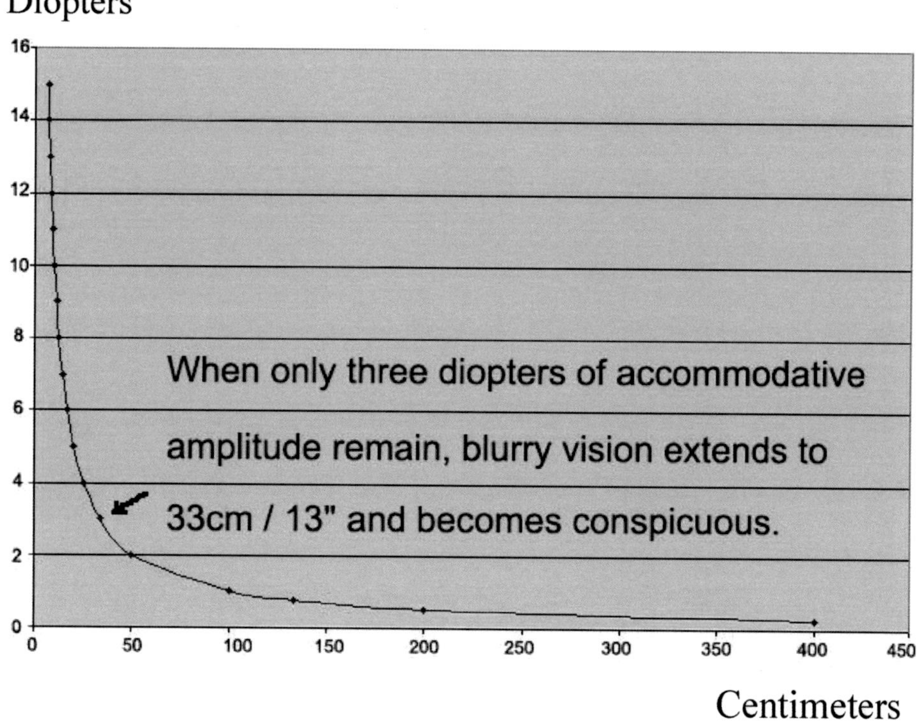


[22] The accommodative range tends to reduce gradually over many years. It usually goes unnoticed in the early stages, especially if there is no need to view anything within 4 to 5 inches (10 to 12.5cm) from the eyes. The loss becomes more noticeable when the amplitude reduces further; diminishing from eight to four diopters which results in blurry small print up

to 5 or 10 inches respectively (13 or 25cm) from the eyes. Presbyopia is generally considered symptomatic when the remaining amplitude is down to three diopters and reading material has to be held beyond 13 inches (33cm) for clarity.[4,14] It is when amplitude falls below two diopters that you will notice your arms have definitely become too short…

Much research has been done to find the cause of presbyopia, yet due to the complex and delicate nature of the eye it is difficult to get an exact picture of how the focusing process works and why it might fail. Subtle changes in an alive and moving target with many variables are difficult to record accurately. Opinions among scientists therefore still vary and contradictions exist between their conclusions.[2,5,14-16]

[21] Various studies say presbyopia is inevitable and cannot be halted or prevented.[2,5,16] One claims it affects 100% of the population over fifty years of age,[2] while another study in Tanzania which included 900 people over fifty shows a prevalence of barely 70%.[17]

An interesting finding from the Tanzania study is that those living in villages with a predominantly outdoor lifestyle (herders and farmers) have only one third the prevalence of presbyopia than their counterparts (small shopkeepers) living in town. This significant difference appears to oppose a claim that solar radiation contributes to presbyopia.[6]

[20] A contributory cause that is often cited is that the lens continues to grow with age. New cells are constantly added to the outer layers of the lens, while old cells in the center remain in place. One theory of presbyopia is that these older cells are

compressed in the core of the lens, causing a hardening of the nucleus which increasingly reduces the ability of the lens to change shape for near focus.

Due to this process of the lens growing and hardening with age, you may have been told that there is nothing that can be done to prevent presbyopia from happening, and that reading glasses will be a permanent fixture in your life from about age forty onwards. Oddly enough, the presumed hardening of the lens does not happen to everyone.

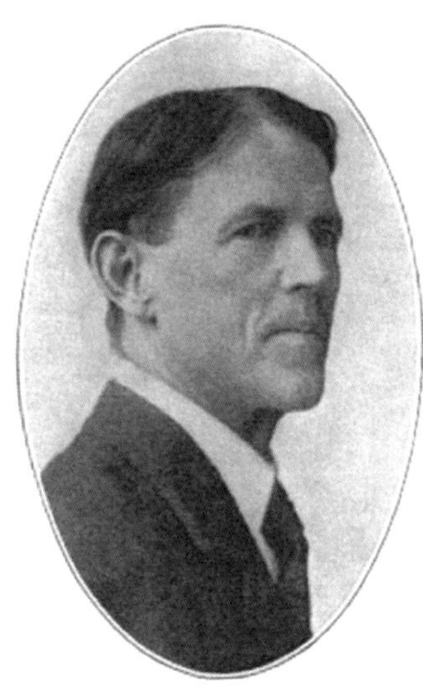

*W. H. Bates, M.D.*

In his early fifties, Dr. William H. Bates, an eye surgeon from New York, was told that his lenses were "hard as stone" and that no one could do anything for him. He did not believe this theory of the lens hardening, and set out to prove that he could regain his near vision. It took him about six months to be able to read a newspaper again without glasses, and a year to completely regain his ability to focus at four inches, but he said that after curing himself, it never took that long to cure anyone else.[18]

I often hear from people that as soon as they started using reading glasses or bifocals their vision at the near point rapidly declined. Texts that they were still able to read without glasses became blurry too, and their dependency on glasses increased.

Research actually confirms that the first use of reading glasses causes a decline in near vision focus.[19] This obviously is not the path you want to take or to continue on. But what can be done to avoid the slippery slope of worsening vision as you age?

Thankfully, Dr. Bates developed an easy-to-use method to keep or regain near vision. Regardless of your age and current prescription, your ability to read small print does not need to be lost forever.

[19] In our modern society, written words are useful to us in so many ways. From six or seven years of age when we first learn to read, to college text books, novels, newspapers, and myriad other forms of printed pages, as well as endless information coming to us on electronic screens, reading continues to educate, entertain and inspire us. It is no wonder that we hate to give it up when our eyes no longer want to focus.

We would much rather squint, strain, or use glasses than give up on reading! The bad news is that squinting, straining and using glasses cause progressively worse eyesight. The good news is that we can use each reading task as an opportunity to naturally improve near vision.

[18] Whether your blur is so advanced that you currently need 3.00 diopter or stronger reading glasses, or whether you have just begun to experience blurry vision at close range, reading can help reduce that blur, if you know how to use it well.

**Reading is to the mind what exercise is to the body. As by the one, health is preserved, strengthened and invigorated; by the other, sight, imagination and mental efficiency are enormously improved.**[20]
William H. Bates, M.D.

You probably guessed it by now: your blurry vision has little or nothing to do with your arms shrinking... So what is the real cause of your inability to focus close-up?
The next chapter explores this with you and prepares you for the book's main purpose: to overcome one more person's need for the crutches that are reading glasses.

# Step 1. Meet Your Blurry Vision

[17] Now that you want to improve your near vision, it is well worth exploring the things you do that tend to lead to blurry vision. Awareness of negative influences is very useful when you wish to change to new, positive ways.

Dr. Bates realized that both mental and physical strain affects your eyes, and the two are interconnected. As an example of this link, looking at something unpleasant may make you pull up your nose, wrinkle your forehead and narrow your eyelids. Look away from this object and the physical strain will reduce, but it will likely not go completely until you stop thinking about what you saw.

[16] You may not be consciously aware of how you strain your eyes either mentally or physically, so I will give a few examples. Can you identify with any of the following strain sources?

- **Making an effort to see better**. Any effort made to see better will create more blur in the long run. Try each of these forms of visual effort to check whether they cause better or worse vision for you.

  - **Squint** or physically try hard to focus. With squinting or narrowing your eyelids you may notice an increase in clarity. You may think this is 'working well' for you as it allows you to read without glasses. Yet the effort required cannot be sustained for long, and when you stop the squint, text often looks even blurrier than before. Squinting is therefore not a long-term solution. By the way, look in a mirror and squint. Would you want to look like this all the time?

- **Stare**: Look at one detail for some time to try see it better. Keep your eyes still; no moving, no blinking. Typically the strain to do this lowers vision within a few seconds.

- **Diffuse**: Attempt to see more than one detail clearly at the same time. The anatomical design of your eyes means this is physically impossible – only one detail can be seen clearly at a time.

- **Test**: Use small print to test your vision in a 'succeed or doom' fashion. Unnecessary failure follows when small print or eye-charts are used in this way.

- **Mental strain,** such as strong emotions, deep sorrow, depression, negative thoughts, dislikes, avoidance issues, worry, fear or pain.

- **Insufficient attention to details** at the near point, or only doing so with glasses. Eye movement is reduced either way and your focusing power diminishes through lack of use.

- Modern **speed reading methods** use techniques contrary to natural vision.
- **Not letting tired eyes close**, or opening them before they feel rested.
- **Insufficient blinking**. Healthy eyes blink every two or three seconds, on average. These blinks are fast, easy, and barely noticeable.
- **Using plus lenses** (reading glasses). Especially glasses that are too strong. My definition of 'too strong' is that you see with perfect clarity through these glasses.
- **Using minus lenses** (for distance vision) while reading within arm's length.
- **Holding the head still** (freezing the neck in place) while reading. Tilting the head back to read is another habitual neck strain. Neck strain contributes to eyestrain and vice versa, so it is best to release those neck muscles!

Chances are that you got to this point of presbyopic vision through straining to see on some level, either physically or mentally, either consciously or not.

Your blurry vision at the near point is simply a sign of strain. As such, the blur can be seen as a messenger. This messenger comes running to you as soon as you strain to read and it yells: "Stop that strain!"

Unfortunately most of us do not hear this message at all. Instead we listen to a message that is imposed by our culture. It says, "You are over forty. What do you expect? Get your eyes checked – you probably need reading glasses."

You may stubbornly refuse the glasses and get by with squinting and staring for as long as you possibly can, but the incredible eyestrain this creates can jeopardize your distance acuity as well as your near vision, and defeats the purpose. So, sooner or later, you get glasses, which silence the messenger. The real message can now be ignored, until the strain worsens and the glasses are no longer strong enough…

Yes, glasses allow you to read, but they do nothing to relieve the underlying strain. On the contrary, glasses tend to cause more strain, which is why vision usually declines rapidly when people start to use them. Within a few weeks, you may find that you can no longer read larger print without glasses that so recently was still within your range.

Researchers at the University of California at Berkeley studied the effect of the first pair of reading glasses given to people aged 21 to 44. Participants were asked to use +1.50 diopter glasses for all near vision tasks, such as computer use and reading, for two months. On average the glasses were used 3.5 hours per day. At the end of the two months twenty-six of the thirty participants had lost an average of two-thirds of a diopter in accommodative range. For the next two months the reading glasses were not used at all, yet these people did not recover their original near focus ability. This study rightfully concluded that it would be best to delay the prescription of reading glasses.[21]

Glasses have a focal center in each lens through which the eye sees best. The further away from the optical center you look through the lens, the less clarity it provides. This results in an unnatural tendency to keep the eyes centered which demands an unnatural amount of head motion to replace eye motion, or you simply squint more when looking through the sides. Either way adds strain.

Looking through glasses also distorts the size, form and color of everything seen, which takes some getting used to. As a rule, the eyes go from bad to worse when using glasses. Keep this in mind next time you habitually reach for them.

After Dr. Bates cured his own presbyopic eyes in his early fifties,[22] so many patients who were unable to read without glasses recovered, that he felt most, if not all, can be cured.[23]

**What to do about glasses?**
Throwing your glasses out is a good start. Sometimes complete avoidance of glasses is all that is required to return to natural clarity, yet most people need additional guidance and help before glasses can be discarded forever. Dr. Bates recommended not using glasses at all. Minimal use of lower strength glasses is another option which allows for progress but this extends the time it takes to get to clarity.

**Discard Glasses**
Easy to say, something else to do. But it is a fact that no one can be cured without glasses and wear glasses at the same time. I know how difficult it is from personal experience. It required a year before I was convinced that my eyes could not be cured unless I stopped wearing glasses. I could not wear them even for emergencies without suffering a relapse.

Patients who are really anxious to be cured can discard glasses and obtain benefit almost from the start. Wearing of glasses becomes s fixed habit. The idea of going without them is a shock. The honest determination to do all that is possible to be done for a cure makes it easy or easier to discard glasses at once. People tell me that after they have discarded their glasses for a few days they do not feel as uncomfortable as they expected.[24]

William H. Bates, M.D.

[15] If your glasses give you perfect clarity – they are too strong and will be impediments to improving your vision. As you want to read with your 'bare' eyes again, you will have to give your eyes the opportunity to relax out of their current level of strain. Not using glasses at all, or only using lower-strength glasses when needed, gives your vision the necessary room for improvement, and a reason to relax into clarity.

I suggest that you do all the activities described in this book without your glasses, and that you accept your blurry vision as a friendly reminder to relax into seeing better. Think of it this way: you may as well enjoy your blurry vision while it lasts, because it will not be with you for much longer! When you stop trying to see better, better vision comes to you.

*********************

Not using glasses at all, or only using lower-strength glasses when needed, gives your vision the necessary room for improvement, and a reason to relax into clarity.

*********************

For paragraphs that you cannot yet read, use glasses that are a quarter or half diopter lower than your regular glasses. Some people even like to step down by three quarters or a whole diopter. If your optometrist is not helpful in this respect, switch to a behavioral optometrist.[25] Alternatively, cheap 'readers' are available in many stores, or more personalized glasses can be bought affordably online.[26] When you can read easily with these lower-strength glasses, it is time to step down another quarter diopter or more.

**Bifocal, multifocal or progressive lenses**

If your presbyopia has progressed to the point that even distance vision is affected, your doctor may have prescribed bifocal, multifocal or progressive lenses. These lenses have a different diopter (power) in the upper half of the glasses. In the case of presbyopia, the upper part will be a lower strength plus lens, while in the case of myopia (nearsightedness) combined with presbyopia, the lower part of the lens has a lower strength minus lens. The latter group can usually still read easily without glasses, yet taking glasses off regularly is a nuisance (or taking contact lenses out for reading is impractical) so they resort to bifocals.

Bifocal and multifocal lenses add to your visual strain by adding neck strain (see *Posture* in Step 2, page 38) and are therefore worse for your vision than regular lenses.

In the case of presbyopic multifocal glasses it is best to return to single vision lenses and take the glasses off for distance vision. Your distance vision will be the first to improve when your eyestrain diminishes.

In the case of myopic multifocal glasses it is also best to return to single vision lenses and take the glasses off for reading. If you use bifocal contact lenses a solution can be to switch to reduced prescription single vision contact lenses instead. Either way, I suggest you learn the Bates Method and regain clear vision for all distances.

**Pinhole Glasses**

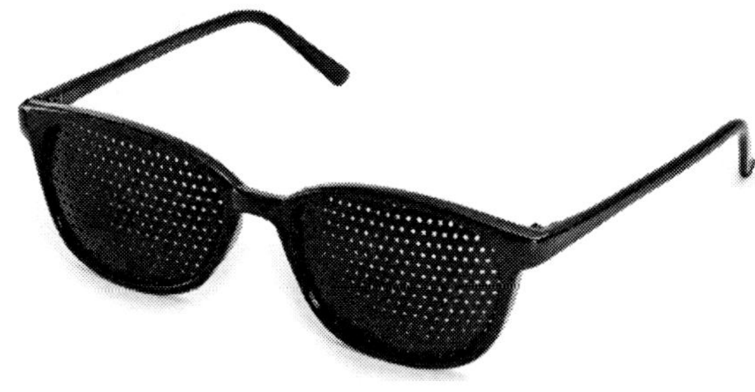

Instead of reading glasses, many people find they can use pinhole 'glasses' for extra clarity when needed. Pinhole glasses do not actually have any glass in them; they are made of black plastic with small holes to see through. Pinholes restrict light rays to central rays only. These rays do not get refracted (bent) by your eye's lens and therefore provide a clear image to the retina. In bright enough light pinhole glasses can be a useful transition tool that reduces the need for 'readers' or prescription glasses. Pinhole glasses are available from my website.[27]

Lili, one of my students who had presbyopia, told me she used modified pinhole glasses for driving. She knew that driving is not advised at all with pinhole glasses (they restrict the visual field far too much) but she found a solution for this problem. She cut out the top half of the black plastic 'lens' so she could see distance unrestricted through this upper gap while she could also read the car's gauges through the bottom half with the pinholes.

**Presbyopia can be avoided**

Not everyone develops presbyopia in their forties. In fact, some people keep their good vision well into their seventies and eighties and never need reading glasses.

Dr. Bates came across numerous people like that. He gave the following example of what can happen when someone recognizes early on that strain is the problem and then takes appropriate action.

A man of sixty-five, examined in a moderate light indoors, was found to have a vision of 20/10. In other words he could see twice as far as the normal eye is expected to see. He also read diamond type* at less than six inches, and at other distances, to more than eighteen inches.

In reply to a query as to how he came to possess visual powers so unusual at his age, or, indeed, at any age, he said that when he was about forty he began to experience difficulty, at times, in reading. He consulted an optician who advised glasses. He could not believe, however, that the glasses were necessary, because at times he could read perfectly without them.

The matter interested him so much that he began to observe facts, a thing that people seldom do. He noted, first, that when he tried hard to see either at the near-point or at the distance, his vision invariably became worse, and the harder he tried the worse it became. Evidently something was wrong with this method of using the eyes.

Then he tried looking at things without effort, without trying to see them. He also tried resting his eyes by closing them for five minutes or longer, or by looking away from the page that he wished to read, or the distant object he wished to see. These practices always improved his sight, and by keeping them up he not only regained normal vision but retained it for twenty-five years.

"Doctor," he said, in concluding his story, "when my eyes are at rest and comfortable, my vision is always good and I forget all about them. When they do not feel comfortable I never see so well, and then I always proceed to rest them until they feel all right again."[28]

* See page 90 for an explanation of diamond type.

**Step 1 Summary – Meet Your Blurry Vision**

✓ Blurry vision is caused by physical and mental strain.

✓ Blurry vision is a message that points to your level of strain.

✓ Glasses silence the messenger and cause more strain over time.

✓ Not using glasses, or using lower-strength glasses only when needed, will allow your vision to improve.

✓ Avoiding bifocal or multifocal lenses will aid your progress.

✓ Accept your current blurry vision and stop trying to see better.

✓ Presbyopia can be avoided by rest.

## Step 2. Time for a Good Rest

[17] It is time to let go of strain! You have probably been trying to fight the blur; you have likely tried hard to see better through squinting and straining to see, but at best your vision improves only temporarily when you do that. It is time to switch tactics, and start releasing the strain that has built up.

Bates said that presbyopia is cured just as any other error of refraction is cured: by **rest**. Some people are cured quickly, even in as short a time as fifteen minutes, others are slow, but as a rule relief is obtained within a reasonable time.

In one case a man was cured simply by closing his eyes for half an hour. His wife was cured in the same way, and when Dr. Bates saw the couple six months later they had had no relapse. Both had worn reading glasses for more than five years.[29]

[16] To make fast progress to clarity you want eyes that are truly rested. It is time to explore several ways of achieving visual rest.

Take off your glasses. Place the medium chart (pages 129-131) at a distance where the top six lines are easily readable. This might be ten or fifteen feet away. Then:

- [15] Close your eyes and cover them with the palms of your hands. This is called palming. Rest your elbows on a pillow, table, or chair backrest. Keep your hands slightly cupped to avoid applying pressure on your eyelids.

  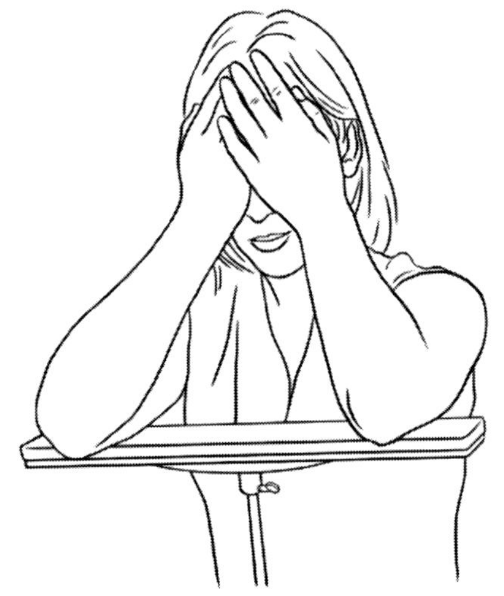

  Notice if there is any tension in the muscles of your face, especially right around the eyes, and see if you can let go of some or all of that tension. Listen to relaxing music and let your mind drift to pleasant thoughts while your eyes rest.

- While palming your eyes, imagine that you are looking at a familiar scene that you like. View it from a distance where you easily see it clearly. Look around with ease and interest and notice lots of details and colors. Notice how your eyes feel when you imagine this.

- Now imagine a tennis ball or a similar small ball rolls into the scenery. Approach it. Pick it up. Softly touch it with your fingers; explore its texture. Notice its colors and details. Slowly bring it closer to your eyes and enjoy seeing or imagining even more details. Imagine that the ball floats slightly up from your hands and moves in various directions with a gentle easy motion.

  If you start to feel any tension in your eyes or your head, release this strain before returning your attention to the ball.

- If you find it difficult to clearly imagine this ball, replace it with something that you can imagine easily.

- Then remove your hands while you keep your eyes closed for another minute. Check in with your face muscles, your posture and your breathing. Do you feel more relaxed?

- When your eyes have adjusted to the light on your closed eyelids, briefly open your eyelids, less than a second, just long enough to 'take a photograph' of whatever is in front of you. Quickly close your eyelids again and notice how the image you saw is still in your brain and you may remember some of its details for a while.

  Turn your head and briefly open your eyelids to take a new 'photograph'. Notice how you don't need to *do* anything for an image to appear in your mind.

  Seeing is meant to be effortless like this; a series of 'photographs' flashing into your brain, instantly ready for you to interpret them. It is as if you see from the back of your head, not consciously using your eyes at all. You simply let light come in.

  The less effort you make to see, the less muscle tension pulls the eyeball out of shape. The image in your mind will therefore be clearer. You can relax into seeing.

- Open your eyes and let them blink as much as they want. Can you keep this sense of effortless seeing? Can you let light and images come in, as they are, without wanting to change how they come in? Is the medium chart easier to read now?

Practice this effortless way of seeing:

- Look at the chart and pick a letter you like. Close your eyes for ten seconds while you imagine this letter even clearer. Alternate that with opening your eyes for a flash to check the letter. Do this without effort; no 'trying' to see the letter, just look at it briefly each time.

- Look at objects around you. Notice the colors. Which color do you like best? Close your eyes for a count of ten and remember your favorite colors, one at a time. Open your eyes for two seconds and check these items. Repeat several times.

Palm often and for as long as you like. Especially in the first few weeks, intersperse all reading with brief periods of palming or closing your eyes. Palm a few seconds or a few minutes every hour. A longer session of half an hour or more usually brings even better results.

My own longest palming session lasted six hours and made the biggest difference in clarity because I reached a much deeper level of relaxation than I do in a few minutes.

**Two levels of strain**

When vision first becomes blurry it is a sign that some eye muscles are under strain. The typical initial reaction to this blur is to make some effort to see better. This effort produces a second layer of strain, usually in the eyelids and facial muscles. Squinting soon becomes a habit. Squinting may bring back some clarity, yet the added strain of squinting, and therefore the clarity, is not sustainable.

When you begin to release strain, the first level of relaxation dissolves this outer layer of strain created by squinting. Unfortunately, the result can be a temporary increase of blur. Not everyone experiences a temporary increase in blurry vision, but some students get discouraged by it and abandon the method before it has a chance to produce real results. If this happens to you, don't give up! You have to accept that you need to let go of the 'false clarity' obtained by squinting. Real and sustainable clarity comes only when you let go of the deeper original strain. You need to reach that deeper level of relaxation.

Palming will help you find both levels of strain so you can begin to release them. The more you palm and the longer your sessions, the sooner you will become familiar with deeper levels of relaxation. It is good to get yourself to the point where just thinking about palming relaxes your eyes.

**The cure of imperfect sight can only be accomplished without effort. Too many patients believe that the cure of imperfect sight is very complicated, and that they have to make a great effort. It is only when they become convinced that the one way they can obtain perfect sight is by rest, that a permanent improvement is obtained.**[30]

William H. Bates, M.D.

When you no longer allow your eyes to become strained for any reason, you will see the best results.

[16] **Sunlight**

Squinting against bright light is a common contributor to eyestrain. Yet, in essence, your eyes are light-finders and sunlight is their reason for being. Sunlight is a key nutrient that supports the health of your eyes. Without sunlight, the body will suffer from 'mal-illumination;' it may become prone to infections and diseases and the eyes become sensitive to light.

Dr. John Ott, a photographer and cinematographer, used time-lapse photography to show the effects of fluorescent and color lights on plants, animals and humans. He found that the limited spectrum of artificial lights caused various bio-chemical changes and resulted in a variety of health challenges depending on which part of the spectrum was missing. When the missing range of the spectrum was supplemented or sunlight was used, these health challenges disappeared. Ott concluded that the full spectrum of wavelengths, from infrared through ultraviolet, is required for optimal health.[31]

As a result of his research Ott developed full spectrum light bulbs which are now widely available. Although such full spectrum lamps are excellent, actual sunlight is still preferable.

Most glasses, contacts and sunglasses (and actually any glass, including windows) filter out the ultraviolet (UV) portion of the spectrum. Without UV waves the pupil contracts less than it should, thus causing more light to enter the eye. This in turn creates a desire for darker glasses and an increased sensitivity to light.

> **The fear that light will hurt the eyes actually produces sensitiveness to light.**[32]
> William H. Bates, M.D.

To improve vision, your eyes need to be comfortable in all light levels, without the need to be shaded. The solution is to spend more time outdoors without glasses, and use the sunning technique described below to become comfortable in bright light. Within a few weeks the pupil response will be restored, you will no longer feel a need to squint in bright light and regular blinking will be enough to keep your eyes at ease.

I certainly do not recommend staring at the sun in order to overcome any spectrum deficiencies, yet I do recommend that you give your eyes a daily sunbath whenever weather permits. Sunning your eyes is easy and safe to do:

- **Sunning**

  Start with the basic sunning practice when the sun is relatively low in the sky. In summer or near the equator that is within two or three hours of sunrise or sunset while during winter months at high latitudes a noon sun is fine.

  Basic sunning: With your eyes closed, point your nose to the sun. Gently turn your head from side to side and enjoy the warmth and light on your closed eyelids for five to ten minutes. When you are done, keep your eyes closed and turn around so the sun is behind you. Open your eyes, blink, and notice how your eyes feel.

Advanced sunning: When your eyes feel very comfortable during basic sunning you are ready for the next level. Face the sun with eyes closed, then turn your head ninety degrees to the left (chin to shoulder) and open your eyes. Blink often while you slowly begin to turn your head back towards the sun.

Pay close attention to how your eyes feel: as soon as the light seems too bright you will have a tendency to squint. Do not squint: gently close your eyes instead. Keep the eyes closed and complete the head turn to the right shoulder. There you open your eyes and blink back towards the sun, again only to your point of comfort. Close your eyes when the light seems too bright and keep them closed until your chin is at the left shoulder again.

Repeat this process for a few minutes. With daily practice your eyes will become more and more comfortable with bright light. Eventually you will be able to blink softly all the way from side to side. Do not rush this process: stay within your level of comfort, and always blink as your eyes pass through the sun itself.

After sunning: Look at the horizon for a few seconds, then shift your attention to an object within a few feet from your eyes (this can be one of the eye-charts held in your hand). Blink regularly as you alternate from far to near and back.

On cloudy or rainy days you can use a bright lamp (250W or more)[33] as a temporary substitute to keep light sensitivity at bay.

- **Sunning and palming combo**
  Alternate palming and sunning your closed eyes for five seconds at a time. When you go back and forth from darkness to light you gently stimulate and relax the pupil response. Finish with a minute or two of basic sunning.

The more time you spend outside in natural light, the better your eyes will feel. In extremely bright conditions the brim of a hat can be used to shade your eyes if needed.

**It is not light but darkness that is dangerous to the eye. Prolonged exclusion from the light always lowers the vision, and may produce serious inflammatory conditions.**[34]
William H. Bates, M.D.

## [15] **Massage & Acupressure**

The key to clear eyesight is physical relaxation of the muscles of the visual system. Besides your focusing muscles, this also includes your eyelid muscles and other muscles near the eyes. The focusing muscles are not usually under your conscious control, but others you can relax more easily. Your eyelids, for example, will release tension as soon as you think about them. You can easily let go of any strain you feel there. Other muscles around the eyes can be encouraged to release with a gentle massage.

Healthy eyes are open eyes with a relaxed look; they show no frown or squint. When you are able to keep the 'accessory vision muscles' relaxed, it becomes easier to influence the deeper layer of tension in the focusing muscles.

Use two or three fingers of each hand to massage around your eyes. Avoid pressure on the eyeballs themselves; just press on the bones around the eyes and also include your forehead, temples, scalp and cheeks. You may find some sore spots. Gently massage them until the soreness is gone.

For acupressure, use the tips of your fingers to stimulate specific points on the face that are related to vision.[35] The pressure and movement from your fingers will bring circulation to these points and help release tension. Other than checking for the location of the spots while you become familiar with this routine, I recommend you do acupressure and massage with your eyes closed.

This image shows which points to release and which points to stimulate for farsighted and presbyopic eyes.

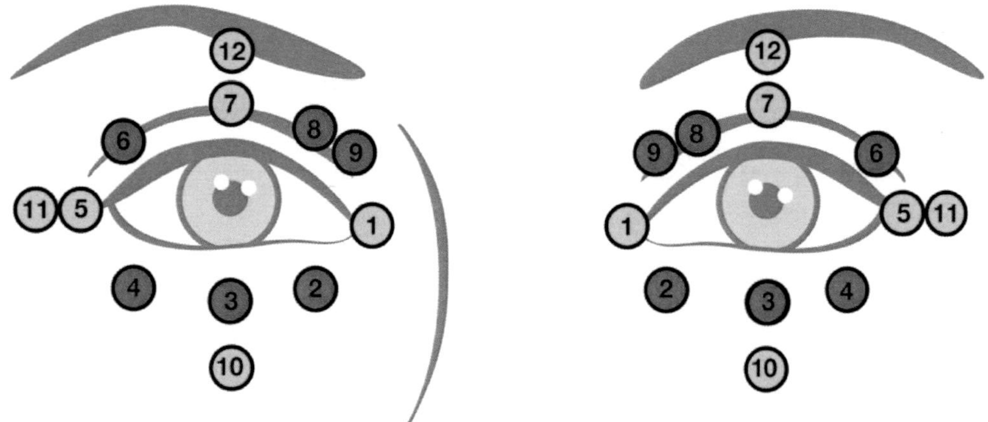


Points 1, 5, 7, 10, 11 and 12 will appreciate being released, as indicated by a blue spot, while points 2, 3, 4, 6, 8 and 9 can be stimulated, as indicated by a red spot. Please use these suggestions as a guide only, and experiment to find what feels best for you.

The points just above the eye (6, 7, 8 and 9) are located on the bone that surrounds the eye. Use your thumb to press upwards against that bone. For points 2, 3 and 4 press gently downwards with your index finger on the bone. Avoid pressure against the eyeball itself.

**To release a point,** you can slowly press the point with your fingertip or thumb while you inhale, and then ease off it as you exhale. Do this for about two minutes on each point, or until any soreness has gone.

**To stimulate a point,** use a small circular massage motion or shake it gently. Do not shake the whole head, only the point itself.

**Posture**
You may find that reading is easier when you look down at a page and that you experience more blur when you hold a book at eye level. This is quite common, perhaps because form follows function. Through daily use, looking down becomes hard-wired for near vision, while looking directly ahead is associated with looking further away. When reading first becomes more difficult, letters are often still clear when viewed with a more downward angle of the eyes. This leads to a tendency to either hold text near the body or to tilt the head back, so the eyes can peer down the nose.

Unfortunately, a habitual overly downward gaze can lead to further visual problems. Optometrist Dr. Elliott Forrest found a strong correlation between prolonged looking down (or tilting the head back) and the development of oblique astigmatism.[36] Bifocal, multifocal and progressive lenses create a similar downward gaze and head tilt; their regular use inevitably leads to astigmatism.[37]

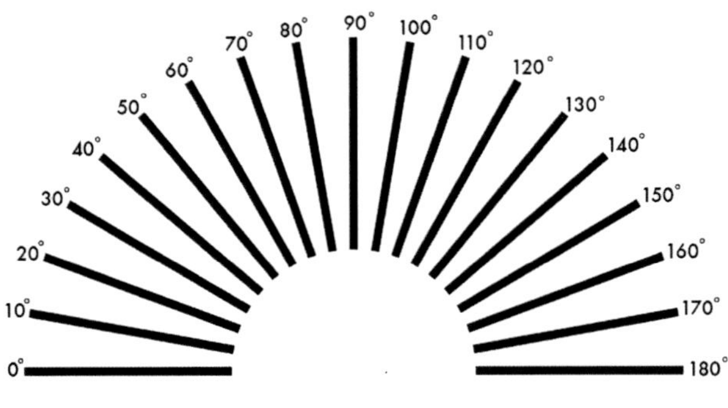


For people who tend to gaze down, Forrest noted that astigmatism develops along 'extorted' axes. This means the right eye's axis is likely to be in the 95-175° range while the left eye's axis tends to be in the 5-85° range. On the other hand, if you habitually peer over your reading glasses and spend more time gazing upward, astigmatism with 'intorted' axes can develop (right eye's axis in the 5-85° range, left eye's axis in the 95-175° range).

Astigmatism results in 'ghost images' or a degree of double vision in each eye. It is a fairly common problem with an estimated prevalence as high as 70%.[38] Forrest's research suggests that astigmatism is preceded by sustained imbalanced use of the extraocular muscles, which are the muscles that move your eyes in all directions.

If you often tilt your head to one side without also tilting your reading material to the same degree you are likely to develop astigmatism at the angle of your head tilt. In addition, tense neck muscles reduce head motion. When you read with less than optimal head motion, your eyes will scan left to right more than natural, and this too can eventually lead to astigmatism. According to Forrest, such side to side eye scanning typically creates horizontal (180˚) astigmatism, which results in blurry vertical lines.

When you begin to practice better visual habits it is obviously beneficial to also practice better posture habits. If you often tilt your head when you read, focus on releasing that neck tension until it no longer occurs. Sometimes a temporary deliberate tilt in the opposite direction can aid a return to balance. The "Close encounters in motion" practice on page 53 is also beneficial in reducing astigmatism.

If you notice ghost images, always check your head position first. Hold text nearer to eye level instead of looking at an angle. Your improved posture will lead to improved vision!

## [15] **The Best Rest**

A good rest goes deeper than merely physical rest; it includes mental rest. When you imagine that you already have clear vision, you foster mental rest. The best mental rest for your eyes comes through combining your imagination with your personal inspiration. A mind at ease increases physical rest, and inspiration then helps to maintain that happy state.

Inspiration is the internal spark that lights your fire of imagination. Let's explore that:

> What motivates you most to improve your vision?
>
> Are you excited at the prospect of seeing clearly again? (I hope so!)
>
> Can you imagine that your vision is perfect again? Right now?
>
> How will you feel when you regain perfect sight?
>
> How brightly will your eyes sparkle with joy?
>
> What will you do when you have clear vision?

Do these thoughts bring a smile to your face? Do they motivate you to take the next step on your path to clarity? Yes? Good! Because your active participation is required to regain clarity. In comparison, glasses are the lazy option, the 'instant fix' that does not require much from you other than placing them on your nose. If you truly plan to ditch the crutches, you need to find your inspiration!

Go ahead; create a clear picture in your mind of the day when you happily throw away your glasses for good, knowing you will never need them again. Sense the joy and freedom this brings, imagine the clarity you see. See yourself taking some action, whether it is effortlessly reading a book without glasses, or kissing a loved one and noticing how his or her face remains sharply in focus.

Keep these things in mind! Replay these positive mental images often, especially on days when your inspiration could do with a little refreshing. When you regularly imagine achieving your goal of reading without glasses, the path toward it becomes a lot easier, no matter how long it takes. Imagine it first; results will follow.

[16] **Remember your successes (things seen perfectly); forget your failures (things seen imperfectly); patients who do this are cured quickly.**[39]
William H. Bates, M.D.

**Step 2 Summary – Time for a Good Rest**

- ✓ Seeing is meant to be effortless.
- ✓ The eyes are subject to two levels of strain. Both need to be released for clear vision to return.
- ✓ Palming creates an opportunity for deep visual relaxation; it releases both levels of strain if done correctly.
- ✓ Blink softly and regularly.
- ✓ Sunlight is essential for eye health.
- ✓ Massage and acupressure stimulate circulation around your eyes.
- ✓ Your posture affects your vision.
- ✓ Positive imagination and inspiration provide mental rest as well as motivation to reach your goal.

# Step 3. Start on Easy Street

[15] When you first stop using glasses or use only lower-strength glasses, make it **easy** on yourself! Use your most favorable conditions to promote relaxation.

- **Light**. If you prefer bright light, use bright light! Sunlight is ideal, yet full spectrum lamps are useful substitutes. Your office supply store or crafts store likely has such lamps available. Examples of lamps to look for are shown on the Visions of Joy website.[40]

- **Distance and size**. Hold text at your optimal distance, wherever you see it best, and choose the smallest print size that is relatively easy for you to read at that distance. Make a note of this distance and letter size (see pages 126-128), so you can check for progress later on.

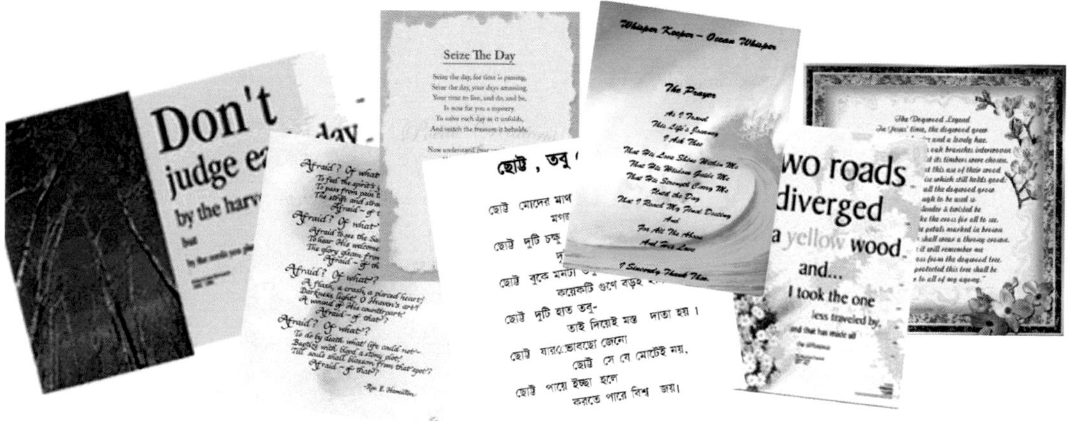


- **Interest**. If at all possible, choose a text that you are interested in! Although you will begin with this book and practice charts, I suggest that for future practice you pick any text that inspires you, perhaps a poem that you love (print it out in a variety of font sizes) or a great book that has you eagerly turning the pages. Your mental focus will greatly aid your physical focus.

- **Use imagination**. From now on, accept your blurry vision as it is in this moment. Don't even *try* to clear it up, as such trying is a strain on the eyes and eyestrain only makes vision worse. Let your imagination fill in the details.

**Important notes on distance**

If you can still read regular print at arm's length, that is a great place to start. To improve your vision at arm's length use steps 4 to 8 alternated with periods of rest, until you can gradually reduce the distance to twelve inches, and then to six.

If your arms are already 'too short,' it is perfectly fine to start your reading practice at ten or twenty feet with a large practice chart (see page 125). It is challenging to improve your near vision if your distance vision is not yet clear, so do check your distance vision with the largest chart first.

If the large chart is not completely clear at a distance of ten feet, use steps 5, 6 and 7 with that chart at ten feet until all lines are easy to read.

When you can easily read the bottom line on the large chart from ten feet, progress to the medium practice chart (pages 129-131) until you easily read all of that from five feet. Here too, use the various steps to clear up any blur before you progress to smaller print nearer to you.

**Fast Improvement Tip**

It is probably easy to relax and read when you hold text at your optimal distance; a point where letters are still seen clearly (point C in the image below). For fast improvement, however, the key is to regularly use your eyes at a distance where they need to relax despite blurry vision. There are two optimal practice distances for overcoming near vision challenges.

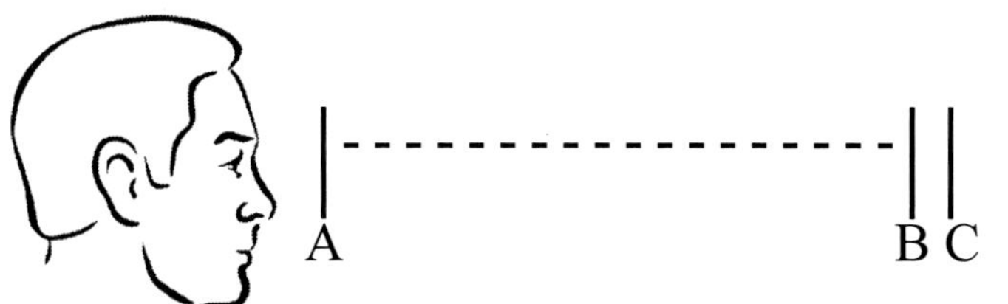


Optimal distances for relaxed reading (C) and for relaxed focus practice (A and B).

Practice Distances:

A = 'Absolutely Impossible'
B = Bit of Blur
C = Clarity

[16] The first distance is just within your blur zone, where letters are only slightly blurry and tend to clear up quickly when relaxed reading habits are used. This is point B. The white halos of steps 7 and 8 will be of great benefit at this distance. If your point B is beyond arm's length you can use pinhole glasses or lower-strength glasses to help bridge the gap.

The second practice distance is within four inches from the eyes, where small print seems impossible to read and you know all effort is useless. This is point A. Motion awareness of step 5 is perfect for use at this distance.

Daily practice at these two distances will ensure that your blur zone (the area between your eyes and point C) will steadily decrease.

Point A can also be used to your advantage if you find your eyes are slow to focus from far to near. When you need to read something after looking at distance, you may find the letters too blurry at first.

The solution is to do the sideways swing within four inches (described in step 5). You thereby simply turn the far to near problem around. Instead of focusing from far to near, you reverse direction and focus from extreme near to normal near, which allows your eyes to focus with much more ease.

You are, of course, free to read at any distance between points A and B, but this area can be a source of frustration and strain. Text appears too blurry to read easily and any benefit from relaxation practices you do is not as instantly evident as it is at point B.

Unless you are good at relaxing with a high degree of blurry vision, I suggest you do most of your reading at point B.

[15] **Optimal nutrition**

Although research has mostly dismissed the impact of nutrition on presbyopia, fluctuations in blood sugar levels can certainly affect your ability to focus, as people with diabetes can attest to. I believe that eliminating artificial sugars from your diet and choosing healthy foods instead can aid your vision improvement.

Staying sufficiently hydrated can also be helpful for your eyes.[41] Drink enough water to have clear (not dark yellow) urine, and minimize alcohol, coffee, black teas and soft drinks which dehydrate you.

Nutrient deficiencies that may be connected to presbyopia are: Vitamins A, B-1, B-2, B-6, C and E, along with glutathione, iron, selenium and zinc.[42-45] A blood test can reveal if any of these nutrients are lacking. If so, rather than take supplements for the rest of your life, include one or more of the relevant food sources in your diet.

[14] This list of whole food sources will help you along. As much as possible choose fresh, local and organically grown plant foods.

**Vitamin A:** dark leafy greens, (kale, turnip greens, mustard greens, spinach, dandelion greens, collards), goji berries, paprika, red pepper, chili peppers, sweet potatoes, carrots, butternut squash, lettuce, apricots, cantaloupe melon, parsley, basil, marjoram, oregano.

**Vitamin B1:** spinach, sunflower seeds, beans, peas, lentils, barley, oats, asparagus, crimini mushrooms, flax seeds, Brussels sprouts, sesame seeds, pine nuts, pistachios, macadamia nuts, pecans, poppy seeds, coriander, sage, mustard seeds, rosemary, thyme

| | |
|---|---|
| **Vitamin B2:** | spinach, almonds, sesame seeds, sun-dried tomatoes, crimini mushrooms, asparagus, soybeans, grains, chili peppers, paprika, coriander, spearmint, parsley. |
| **Vitamin B6:** | sweet potato, sunflower seeds, sesame seeds, spinach, banana, chili peppers, paprika, garlic, pistachios, hazelnuts/filberts, tuna, turkey, beef, chicken, salmon. |
| **Vitamin C:** | hot chili peppers, bell peppers, guavas, kiwis, oranges, tangerines, strawberries, papayas, broccoli, kale, mustard greens, garden cress, cauliflower, Brussels sprouts, thyme, parsley. |
| **Vitamin E:** | spinach, sunflower seeds, almonds, peanuts, paprika, chili peppers, almonds, pine nuts, peanuts, basil, oregano, apricots, tarot root. |
| **Glutathione:** | spinach, broccoli, asparagus, potatoes, peppers, carrots, onion, avocados, squash, garlic, tomatoes, grapefruit, apples, oranges, peaches, banana, melon. |
| **Iron:** | spinach, Swiss chard, squash, pumpkin seeds, beans, lentils, pomegranates, sun-dried tomatoes, sesame seeds, cashews, pine nuts, hazelnuts/filberts, peanuts, almonds, white beans, mollusks, liver, beef, lamb, eggs. |
| **Selenium:** | Brazil nuts, walnuts, sunflower seeds, oats, legumes, tuna, beef, poultry, eggs. |
| **Zinc:** | sesame seeds, pumpkin seeds, squash seeds, watermelon seeds, peanuts, Napa cabbage, palm hearts, green peas, shiitake mushrooms, apricots, peaches, prunes, grapes, bananas, figs, blackberries, raspberries, dates, sun-dried tomatoes, avocados, red meats, crab, oysters. |

**Step 3 Summary – Start on Easy Street**

- ✓ Use your most favorable reading conditions in terms of light, distance, letter size and an engaging topic.
- ✓ Practice most at your optimal distances for fast improvement.
- ✓ Optimal nutrition for your eyes optimizes your chance of success.

# Step 4. Near Vision Warm-Ups

[15] When your near vision became blurry, you probably developed a habit of holding print further out. This is a common tendency, which is practical in the moment, but ultimately not helpful, as your near vision only becomes worse through lack of use. You can increase the reading distance until clarity starts beyond arm's length, at which time you resort to glasses. From then on, chances are that you barely even look at anything within a few inches from your eyes any more, as you do not expect to see it clearly. This is a negative trend which you are about to reverse!

## Palm-Reading

Looking at your own hand is less likely to cause you to 'try to see' than looking at letters would, so it is easier to keep your eyes relaxed while 'palm-reading.'

It is easy to do: Look at the palm of your hand in a relaxed way, blinking regularly. Begin with your arm straight out, and then slowly bring the hand all the way to your nose. Move your hand from arm's length to your nose and back twenty times or more, while observing the details in your palm. This will gently stimulate your eye muscles.

Even this gentle way of using your eyes may at first cause discomfort in the forehead or around your eyes when your hand comes close. If that happens, do not worry; this is a positive sensation which happens when underused muscles are being stimulated. If it is uncomfortable close your eyes and let any soreness dissipate. Then, while your eyes remain closed, imagine that you watch your hand move in and out.

When you can do this without discomfort, continue your practice with open eyes. You may need to close your eyes regularly to avoid discomfort or strain when looking at the near point, yet with daily practice you will soon overcome this.

Also do this palm-reading practice one eye at a time, by covering the other eye with the palm of your other hand. Do not close the covered eye; keep it open and let it blink along with the eye that you use.

If one eye sees better than the other, begin palm-reading with the better eye. If both eyes have a similar level of blur it does not matter with which eye you start. After each eye has had a turn of twenty or more, do another set of twenty or more with both eyes open. As the eye with blurrier vision (if applicable) has had the most recent stimulation it is gently encouraged to play an equal part in vision with both eyes open.

**Close Encounters**

The rest of the day – use your near vision! Notice or imagine the details of anything that comes close to your eyes – the food on your fork as you eat; the rim of your drinking glass; the texture of your pillowcase; the petals of a flower you smell; the face of a person who embraces you, etc. By paying more attention to such daily 'close encounters' you can relearn to use your near vision effortlessly.

Regularly pick up something familiar, preferably something colorful without printed text. It could be a picture, but a 3-D object is even better: a flower, an apple, a cup – anything you like. Bring it to eye level and look at it while your fingers trace over it. Do not strain to see it better; just observe the colors, its shape, and feel its texture and weight. Blink easily and often.

Bring your familiar object even closer to your eyes, to where the details blur. Ignore this blurriness. Instead, remember or imagine how it looks when you see it clearly. Close your eyes and enjoy the memory of clarity, and imagine that you can see this object with the same or even better clarity right now, very close to you. Then open your eyes.

[14] **Close encounters in motion**

Move your familiar object around – left, right, up, down, diagonally, further away, back to your eyes and in any direction you like. Also make some big circular motions around the edge of your peripheral field in both directions. Let all this motion be smooth and keep looking at the various details while you blink and breathe in a relaxed way. Free your neck and let your head move along as needed. Avoid robot-like motion of the head; the eyes and nose are not meant to be in perfect sync! Simply let the head follow the eyes naturally.

Feel free to close your eyes and follow the motion in your mind. Your eyes will respond the same way when closed as when they are open, so either way is good practice of relaxing with near vision.

**As close as your nose**

When you are comfortable with such close encounters, you can even examine the tip of your own nose. When did you last look at your nose without a mirror?!? It is a useful habit to develop, especially as allowing the eyes to converge to this degree requires that you let go of any remaining strain.

**Memory and imagination practice**

This practice is a little more advanced, yet very useful in the early stages. Use both the small and the medium practice charts (see pages 129-133). If your distance vision is blurry, use the medium and large charts instead.

Hang the larger chart on a wall and stand at the distance where you see it best. Look at the top letter R on the large chart on the wall. Now close and cover (palm) your eyes, and remember this R. Alternate looking at the letter R then palm and remember the letter R until your memory of the letter is nearly equal to the sight. If you are unable to remember the whole R you may be able to imagine a small black period as forming part of it, which works equally well in this practice.

Next hold the smaller chart in one hand and a blank piece of paper in the other. Hold both papers at a regular reading distance with your hands a foot (30cm) or more apart, or place both papers on a table in front of you, a foot or more apart.

While still holding the mental picture of the R, look at the blank page. Close your eyes (palm if using a table) and remember the R. Upon opening your eyes look again at the blank page but bring it a little closer to the smaller chart. Gradually reduce the distance between the white page and the smaller chart, until you can look directly at the near letter R and imagine it as well as the distant R you remember. When you succeed, the near R will be clearer and other letters on the near chart will become clearer too.

Using your memory and imagination for better vision is one of the best ways to relax into seeing. Let your mind do the work and let go of all physical effort. If you are not good at remembering, just pretend at first; your ability to imagine and remember will improve with practice.

[13] **Balance your eyes**

When one eye sees better than the other (called anisometropia, which is common with presbyopia[46]), it is good to give the eye with blurrier vision a chance to catch up. There are several ways to achieve visual balance and the methods chosen should ideally be tailored to the individual's specific needs. To stay within the scope of this book I offer two basic practices here that you can easily do on your own.

A common approach is to cover the better eye for a few minutes with an eye-patch. Do any of your favorite practices in this book to encourage the non-covered eye to relax. Use your most favorable conditions and work on the edge of this eye's blur zone as well as at the near point for fast improvement.

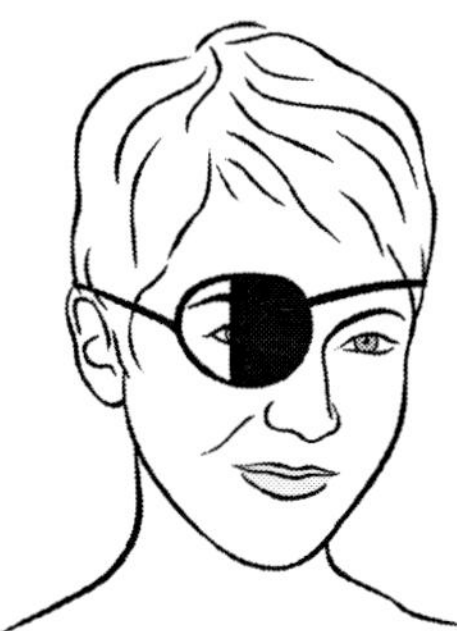

If you are anything like me, the loss of part of the visual field from wearing an eye-patch can be terribly frustrating. For that reason I tend to cut a hole in the patch. This allows the now partially covered eye to take part in seeing, even if only peripherally. This eye remains covered on the side nearest the nose, ensuring that the other eye is called upon to actually focus on the object of your attention.

Another excellent way to improve the sight of one eye is to cover the eye with blurrier vision with the palm of your hand and look at a familiar object with your better eye at a distance where you see it best. Notice the object's details, colors and shape. Now close both eyes and remember the details, colors and shape. While both eyes are closed, switch hands to cover your better eye. Then open both eyes (the better eye now covered) and look again at your object. Ignore the blur and simply remember the details the better eye saw. You may find this improves the image.

With regular practice of eye-balancing techniques both eyes will start to see with equal clarity.

## Step 4 Summary – Near Vision Warm-Ups

- ✓ Enjoy close encounters! Take every opportunity to look at familiar objects near your face. Whether you look at the palm of your hand or the food on your fork, be interested in details without making an effort.
- ✓ Practice your memory and imagination using two charts and a blank page to bridge the gap between clarity at distance and clarity at the near point.
- ✓ Balance your eyes so both see with equal clarity.

# Step 5. Get into the Swing

[13] When vision is normal, the eyes are in constant motion. The majority of eye movements are small, smooth, extremely rapid, inconspicuous and effortless. People with blurry vision, on the contrary, have eye movements that are slower, jerky and made with effort. When you look at a letter and see it blurred, you may be tempted to look at it longer in an effort to see it better. Such staring is a big strain on the eyes, and it is one habit you really want to give up soon.

******************

The majority of eye movements are small, smooth, extremely rapid, inconspicuous and effortless.

******************

How do you regain natural eye motion? Your interest in details is the main mobilizer of your eyes. Your eyes follow your mind: they shift as soon as your attention shifts. It is each shift in attention which makes eye motion effortless. You can let your eyes shift quickly and easily all day long – through attention for details.

It may take some time to get out of the staring habit because you probably do it unconsciously. Luckily, there are six easy tricks you can apply, anywhere and anytime, which can drastically reduce your tendency to stare.

- **Page motion**. The first trick is to move the page. Gentle side to side or circular motion of your reading materials will encourage your eyes to move too, because now their target is in motion, and they will want to follow! The resulting extra eye motion gives an immediate measure of relief from staring, straining and trying to see.

  Whenever you notice your eyes strain, or when blurry vision creeps in, quickly shake it off with some page movement. Half an inch from side to side will do. Half an inch closer and back is also great, and you can combine left to right motion with near to far motion for greater effect.

[14] Continuous and effortless movement is essential to healthy vision, and when you master it you will no longer need to move the page, as your eyes happily shift on their own again.

- **Head motion** is another excellent aid in beating the staring demon. Just move your head slightly, a quarter of an inch from side to side while you read. This can already make the difference between straining to see and reading comfortably. Good posture will help, because that releases neck tension.

  The best way is to let your head follow to the left when your attention and eyes move left, and let your head follow to the right when your eyes move right. Doing the opposite can cause a strain, so let your head follow your eyes.

  Prove it to yourself: purposely hold your head completely still while you read a few paragraphs. Do you notice your eyes feel less at ease? When your neck is loose and your head is allowed to be in motion, even if it moves only slightly, your eyes will feel much better.

- **The sideways swing within four inches**. Hold this page (or any text you want to read) sideways up in front of your eyes, no more than four inches from your face. Accept any blur and simply look from the white edge on the left side of the paper to the white edge on the right. Skim through the vertical lines of text without trying to read. Let your interest be mostly with the white background and just notice the black and white alternate.

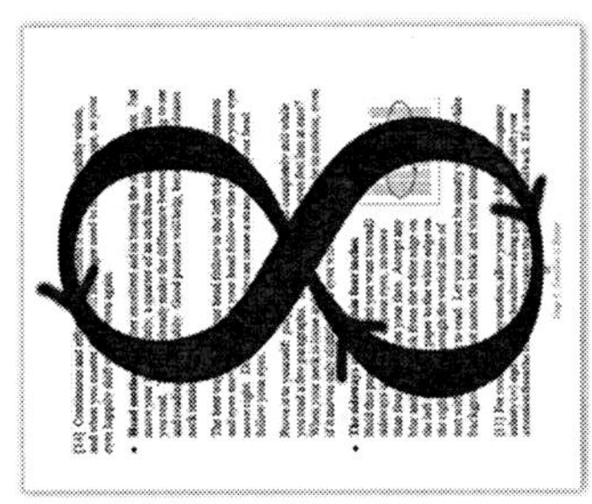

  [13] For continuous easy motion, allow your eyes to follow an imaginary infinity (∞) sign. Let your head move along gently while you shift your attention from the left side of the page to the right side and back. If a circular

or oblong motion seems easier for you, use that instead. The shape does not matter; the key is to let the motion be continuous and effortless. Do make sure the imagined shape is followed in your mind; do not imagine you see it on the page, as the latter creates a strain.

Blink softly, and open your peripheral awareness to include the background around the page. Notice how the page appears to swing from side to side in the opposite direction of your head. Allow this perception of apparent motion to deepen your feeling of relaxation.

Help that sense of motion along by physically moving the page side to side, gently and easily, in the opposite direction to the motion of your head.

For best results keep the page within four inches, do not let it creep away from your eyes.

Do this for three to five minutes (feel free to do more if you like!), and then turn the page right side up and hold it at your normal reading distance. Does the text seem any clearer now?

> [12] Josephine gave herself the gift of a vision lesson for her forty-fourth birthday. I gave her a page of standard-size text to look at, which appeared blurry to her. After practicing the above relaxation technique for five minutes she looked at the same page again, at the same distance, and asked, "Where is the page with blurry print??"
> The text now looked perfectly clear to her.
>
> When Cara (age sixty-eight) first used this technique she noticed it improved her vision too, so she decided to spend more time with it. She relaxed her eyes more and more while she looked at a reading practice card (page 141) held sideways in front of her eyes. After twenty to twenty-five minutes she found she could easily recognize all the letters, while she was still holding the card at four inches!

[14] **Important:** If at any time your eyes feel sore, or you feel any kind of strain around them, close your eyes to rest them until this strain dissipates.

- Next, do a **near-to-far swing**. The aim is to look at print through a range, from clarity to blur and back. Similar to palm-reading this stimulates the eye muscles in a gentle way, as long as you make no effort to see clearly in your blur zone.

<u>Begin at the distance of your best vision</u>.
[13] If clarity begins at three feet or more – hang the medium or large chart on a wall and stand in front of it at the distance where you see it best. Place one foot closer to it than the other, and sway your body gently forwards so the chart is now in your blur zone. Then sway back to the clear zone, and continue going back and forth for several minutes.

If your point of clarity is within arm's length – hold the small or medium chart in your hand and move it back and forth in and out of your blur zone while you simply observe the changes this creates in the print.

Keep blinking and make no effort to clear up the blurry print when it comes close. If you have a tendency to try to see the letters, then let your attention shift over the white background. The idea is to look at the chart with interest, yet without effort.

[14] For variety and enjoyment, do the same near-to-far swing while you look at your favorite photo of a loved one! Or invite this person to actually do it with you… Have fun!

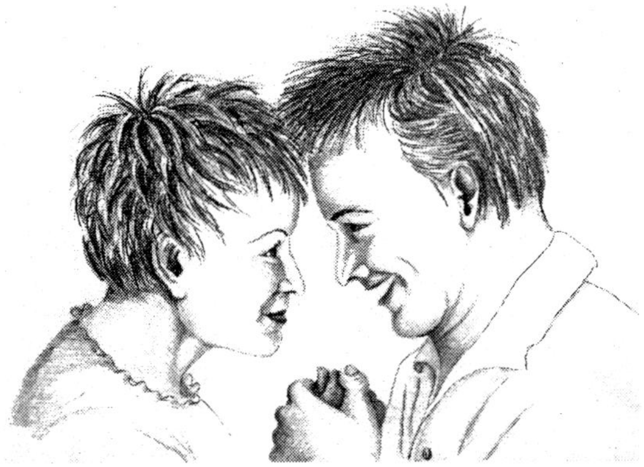

You can also use two charts: a large one on a wall and a small one in your hand. Let your attention shift from a letter on the wall chart to the same letter on the chart in your hand. Continue to shift between the two for five minutes or longer. The constant motion will help release the strain of staring, and you may find the near letters gradually clear up.

- Now do a **letter swing**. Turn your attention back to the large R at the top of the chart. Let your attention shift to the left of the chart and stay aware of the R's location to your right. Next shift to the right of the chart, and notice the R is now to the left of your gaze.

  Be sure to let your eyes and head follow your shifts in attention. Go back and forth for a minute in a smooth easy way. While you do this, imagine that instead of shifting your attention from side to side, the letter swings from side to side. This may be challenging at first, but a little practice will bring results! The trick is to stay aware of the R's location, not its clarity. It may help to continually ask yourself, "Where is the R now?"

  Allow this apparent motion of the letter to continue, and notice that the entire chart swings along. Play with various swing widths and speeds and notice if the perception of the swing reduces tension in your eyes.

  If the R seems to swing easily for you, move down the chart to swing smaller letters. Reduce the width of your side to side shift with the smaller letters. For example, shift from the N to the R in CENTRAL to see the T swing. Your shift should be long enough to get the swing, yet short enough to make it barely noticeable.

  Can you do the letter swing with your eyes closed and remember the chart's motion?

  Can you do this closer to your eyes with smaller letters?

- [13] You are ready for a **universal swing**. Close your eyes and remember (or imagine) the smallest letter o you have ever seen. It may look like this: o or o or even like this o or o.
- Imagine this tiny o with its opening as white as the sun and the outline a solid black. When the white center is as bright as possible, imagine that the letter moves, and that all surrounding objects, no matter how large or small, are moving with it.

  Open your eyes and continue to imagine this universal swing where everything is in motion. This encourages your eyes to shift continuously and smoothly, the way they love to move.

  Alternate imagining the swing with your eyes open with imagining it with eyes closed. When the imagination is just as good with the eyes open as when they are closed, your vision will be much improved!

[14] **Not reading from paper?**

These days, many people read more from computer screens than from paper, and this trend is likely to continue. Unless the screen is small and portable, moving 'the page' is not quite as simple as moving a piece of paper or a book in your hand.

Thankfully, software exists that creates movement on your computer screen. The program is called SwingWindows. You will find a link to a free download at www.visionsofjoy.org.[47]

Alternatively, gently sway your head or upper body a short distance from side to side while you work at a computer. This too will break any tendency to stare. In your peripheral vision the screen will appear to move opposite to your motion. Keep blinking and take regular vision breaks from the screen by briefly looking into the distance or by closing your eyes.

**Step 5 Summary – Get into the Swing**

- ✓ Page motion and head motion encourage relaxed eye motion.
- ✓ Notice apparent motion of objects in your peripheral vision.
- ✓ Use a near-to-far swing: look at details that move in and out of your blur zone.
- ✓ See apparent motion, the universal swing, all day long.

# Step 6. Smaller is Better

[14] The eye's anatomical design allows it to see best in a tiny area right in the center of its field of vision. Peripheral vision (the rest of the visual field) does not have the same high level of clarity as that central point.

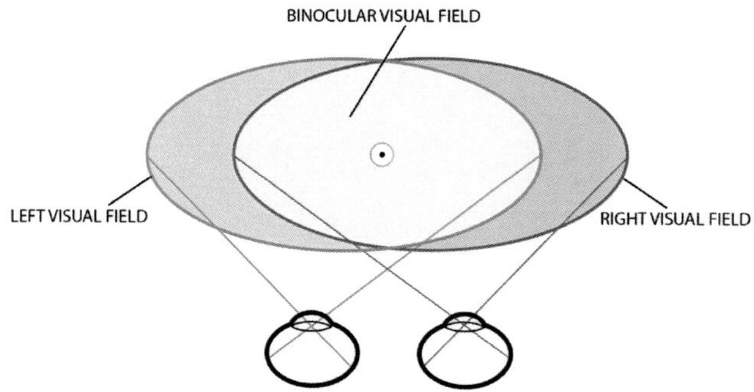


This image resembles your approximate field of vision when both eyes are healthy. The upper edge of your visual field is created by your eyebrows while your cheeks form the lower edge.

The white circle in the center represents the macula region of your retina: an area of relatively clear vision. The black dot within the macula circle represents the point seen by the retina's "fovea centralis," your point of clarity or best vision.

If you try to see clearly with peripheral vision (everything outside of the black dot), you create visual strain. You already know that presbyopia is caused by a strain and cured by rest. Besides the total rest provided by palming (step 2), the eyes are rested through motion (the previous step) and through seeing with central clarity.

The medical term for this is central fixation, and its opposite is eccentric fixation.

*****************

Besides the total rest provided by palming, the eyes are rested through motion and through seeing with central clarity.

*****************

As an eye surgeon, Bates was familiar with these terms and used them frequently. For non-medical doctors, a brief explanation is probably useful.

Central fixation means that the eyes point directly at the detail you want to see and you see that one central detail better than anything else in your view. If you shift your attention away from this detail, even if only slightly, the detail is seen less clearly than when you look at it directly.

If your eyes do not point directly at the detail of interest, or if a peripheral spot is seen better than the detail you look at, you have eccentric fixation.

Bates found that central fixation can be obtained with practice. For people with presbyopia he recommended to start at ten or twenty feet with a regular eye chart.

So let's begin there, and then gradually practice closer to the eyes.

- Place the medium practice chart at ten feet. If the 10 line is not easily read from ten feet, use the largest practice chart at fifteen or twenty feet.

- Begin with a tall posture and let breathing happen naturally and effortlessly. Blink regularly (at least once per line) and close your eyes or palm to rest them as much as needed, which is probably more often than you think!

- Use a relaxed 'let-it-be' attitude rather than 'trying' to see clearly.

- Notice the 'building block' to the left of the top letter R. How many of these blocks did it take to make the R? Take a guess!

  While you count building blocks, notice that whichever part of the R you look at, this part is seen blacker and more distinct than the rest of the letter. When you look at the bottom left of the R, the top right is not seen with the same clarity. True?

If this does not seem to be true for you, close your eyes and think of a black object you have seen and keep your eyes closed until they feel rested. When you open your eyes again, notice that the blackest part of the letter is the part you pay attention to. The rest of the letter will seem slightly less black or less distinct.

If it still does not appear that way, turn it around: instead of imagining that you see the central point best, imagine you see the periphery less distinctly. *Allow* the parts of the chart you are not looking at to be less clear. This will take any effort out of seeing the central part clearest, and that will help create effortless central clarity for you.

- When you are able to see part of the largest letter best, progress to smaller letters and do the same; see or imagine part of each letter blackest and most distinct and the rest of the letter less clearly.

- To ensure that both eyes make progress, cover one eye at a time while observing that you see best right where you look. Allow vision to be less sharp all around this point of central clarity.

- When each eye is able to see part of a small letter better than the rest of that letter, move closer to the chart to where you easily see the period in the bottom line of the chart. Imagine this period best and blackest when your attention is on it, and then look away from the period at letters near it, while you notice that the period is now seen less clearly.

  You may have to shift a few letters away at first to see the period worse. Then slowly progress to the letter right next to the period while still seeing the period less clearly than you do when your attention is directly on it.

- [14] When your central clarity at your optimal distance has improved to the level of seeing the period less clearly when you look right next to it, it is time to notice central clarity closer to your eyes.

  Begin again with the large letter R on the medium chart, and have that chart close enough to see it slightly blurry yet easily readable. Notice that part of the large letter is blacker and more distinct than the rest of the letter that you are not looking at.

- Gradually progress to noticing one part blackest in smaller letters at this distance. When that is easy, bring the chart closer, perhaps one inch at a time, and repeat this practice of central clarity awareness.

- [13] Apply the same technique at the near point with the smallest practice chart (page 133) or with the dot in the center of this number matrix.

  When you cover one eye with the palm of your hand and look at the center dot, what do you see best? The dot or any one of the surrounding numbers? If you see the dot best, you see with central fixation.

  0987654567890
  098765434567890
  09876543234567890
  0987654321234567890
  0987654321•1234567890
  0987654321234567890
  09876543234567890
  098765434567890
  0987654567890

  If you see one of the numbers better than the dot, shift to that number and notice how the dot loses some clarity.

- To improve your central clarity, start to notice small details while allowing peripheral vision to be less distinct. Observe the size of the pupil in someone's eye and notice the eyebrow is a little fuzzy. Check which direction hairs grow in an eyebrow and notice the pupil is now less clear. Go smaller: watch for gradual color changes in a flower petal; see the weave of fabric in clothing. Imagine details everywhere present themselves eagerly to your rapidly moving attention. At all times, notice finer details, both near and far.

### [14] **Beware of the Tunnel Vision Trap**

Even though your best clarity is in the center of your field of vision, please do not fall into the trap of tunnel vision. Your peripheral vision will never be as clear as that central point of clarity, but it is every bit as important! When you lose peripheral awareness and become lost in tunnel vision, the strain on your eyes increases.

Always keep a relaxed awareness of your surroundings, even while you read. This not only reduces strain, it also promotes brief yet crucial glances away from the text – restful mini-breaks for your eyes.

### TV is not for Tunnel Vision

It is even more important to stay aware of your peripheral vision while you watch television, use a computer or use any back-lit screen. Such screens provide the additional challenge to your eyes of having to focus on pixels of light. Converging, which means pointing your eyes at the details you wish to see, is not any harder on a screen, but focusing at the right distance is not as easy when you look into a pixel of light rather than at a paper surface. The information your brain gathers from peripheral vision allows it to compare your distance from the screen to the distance of nearby solid objects so it can better estimate the required focal distance. Dimming your screen can also alleviate some of the stress on your eyes.

### E-readers

With rapidly advancing technology causing a profusion of new electronic devices to appear on the market each month, chances are that you use one or more gadgets with a digital screen, and you may be curious about its use for extended reading. Most of these devices have back-lit screens that create the same vision challenges as computer and TV screens do – they therefore require your vigilance to stay visually relaxed.

Some e-readers use a different display technology; they provide a reading experience that more closely resembles reading from paper. Such "E-Ink" screens are easier on your eyes, especially under natural or bright light.

The option to easily enlarge or reduce font sizes on electronic screens is a useful bonus. Larger text may increase your reading time without glasses, and you can make even better use of this resizing possibility by creating your very own fine print for relaxation practice (see Step 9).

For now, while you are still learning to keep your eyes relaxed, back-lit screens can be a challenge to your sight, and temporarily reducing their use may accelerate your progress to clarity. When you do use them, keep blinking softly, stay aware of peripheral vision and motion (see page 62), adjust screen brightness and text size to your preferred levels, and take plenty of breaks.

**Step 6 Summary – Smaller is Better**

- ✓ Your central vision is your only point of total clarity; peripheral vision is not seen as clearly.
- ✓ A mental attention for details while staying aware of your whole field of vision is in accordance with nature's design of your eyes.

# Step 7. Holy Halos!

[13] You have probably never given it much thought, but the surface of a printed page has much more white space than it has black ink. This fact can be used to your advantage.

When you look at black letters, you are inherently tempted to focus on them and make an effort to see them better. In contrast, looking at white spaces is more restful; there is no such need to focus on white with effort. Therefore, to improve the whiteness of the page by imagining the white spaces to be perfectly white is a lot easier to accomplish than improving the appearance of black letters. The happy side effect of doing so is… exactly: blacker letters!

Look at the white spaces on this page. Do you see variations in the brightness of white? If so, which areas seem whiter? To me, the margins appear duller than the white in and around the letters. You may need to hold the page at your best distance and use a bright light to see this difference.

Anyone with good vision sees or imagines the white spaces in and around letters as white, even whiter than they really are, whereas you may currently see these spaces gray, blurred or indistinct. There is no gray printed there. Unless a pencil-wielding toddler got hold of this page first, the gray exists only in your mind, not in reality. So let's change what is in your mind, and see what happens in reality.

Practice with this page or any text you like, and let your attention roam around the white spaces on the page. Look at the edge of the page, check the margins, follow the white strips between the lines of text, and notice the white spaces between and inside the letters.

Now close your eyes and imagine these white spaces to be perfectly white. Remember them one at a time and let these white spaces be extra white in your mental picture of them. Then open your eyes, look at the white, and remember how white you just imagined it to be.

Repeat that a few times. Your eyes will relax more when there is no need to focus on letters, and the overall appearance of the page is likely to improve.

You may begin to notice something rather peculiar… 'halos' around letters:

- Look at the letter O on the fourth line of the medium practice chart. Hold it at a distance where you see it best and under optimal light. Maybe you notice that the white inside the letter O appears to be whiter than the white of the rest of the chart. Do you notice that the O also seems to have a thin 'halo' of brighter white around it? This illusion of a halo appears because the mind interprets white as whiter when it is right next to black due to the contrast the black provides.

  If you do not yet see a brighter white halo, close your eyes and think of something that is pure white, such as sun-lit fresh snow, bright white paint, or any clear memory you have of a bright white surface. Relax into that memory of pure white for half a minute or longer.

  Open your eyes for a second and imagine this dazzling bright white in and around the O. Alternate several minutes between resting with eyes closed and briefly opening the eyes while you imagine the halos are present and brightly white. Do this in a very relaxed way, with zero effort, until you can imagine or see the white much whiter than before.

- When you are able to imagine the bright white halo in and around the letter O, can you imagine that you see similar halos in and around other letters on the chart?

*The better the imagination of halos, the better the sight.*

- When you can easily imagine halos, bring the chart closer, to just within your blur zone. Accept this blur as your friendly messenger; let it be there. Bring your awareness to how your eyes feel and allow them to remain relaxed. Blink effortlessly, and shift smoothly across the page. Let your attention be mostly with the abundant white spaces of the page and the halos of the letters, which will encourage your eyes to focus without effort.

  To avoid the temptation to look at the black print, pretend that you are a paper quality expert. You are extremely interested in the texture of the white page and could not care less about the black ink added by the printer… Does this new perspective change your view?

- Return to this page and let your attention glide across this string of O's:

  o o o o o o o o o o o O O O O O o o o o o o o o o o

  Remember: accept any blur. Just look at the white in and around the O's and allow your eyes to shift smoothly back and forth along this line.

- [12] Shift your attention from the halos in the string of O's to the halos of the letters on the medium practice chart and back a few times. Pay attention only to the halos.

- Now pick up the near vision chart (the small practice chart) and hold it about four to six inches from your face. Accept the blur. Just look at the white between the lines and allow your eyes to shift easily across the white spaces.

  Your feeling of relaxation is most important at this point. Stay aware of how your eyes feel; let go of any strain or any attempt to see letters blacker. This may result in more blur at first. That is okay. Simply stay as relaxed as possible. You can always look away to avoid strain. Look far enough away and long enough for the eyes to relax. Gradually return to looking nearer until you can look at the white spaces in and around letters with ease. When you relax to a deeper level, your vision improves for all distances.

- After a few minutes of relaxing with the halos close-up, return to the medium chart and hold it just within your previous blur zone. Does it seem easier to read now?

  You know that the letters are printed with black ink, so imagine that they are black, rather than the gray fuzz they may appear to be. This will be easiest when you imagine brighter white halos.

[13] **TIP**:
You will find that, every step of the way, your memory and imagination are your greatest allies in improving your vision. When you test your sight by reading small letters, you tend to fail because you make an effort. When you test your imagination, you are much less likely to strain. You can look at a white wall, then close your eyes, and imagine you see a white surface. Improving on its whiteness is a mere matter of applying some imaginary bright white paint! Transferring that same ease and imagination of white to the halos around letters is a simple trick of the mind. As long as no effort is used, you will soon be able to imagine bright white spaces there too.

## HALOS

by William H. Bates, M.D.

[14] "The eyes, when reading perfectly,
do not look directly at the letters,
but at the white spaces or the halos."[48]

[12] When people with normal sight look at the large letters on the Snellen test card, at any distance, from twenty feet to six inches or less, they see, at the inner and outer edges and in the openings of the round letters, a white more intense than the margin of the card. Similarly, when they read fine print, the spaces between the lines and the letters and the openings of the letters appear whiter than the margin of the page, while streaks of an even more intense white may be seen along the edges of the lines of letters.

It can be demonstrated that this is an illusion. We do not see illusions; we only imagine them. When the white spaces between the lines appear whiter than the margin of the page, we call these white spaces "halos."

These "halos" are sometimes seen so vividly that in order to convince people that they are illusions it is often necessary to cover the letters, when they at once disappear.

Most of us believe we see them, and it is very difficult for many people to realize that the halos are not seen, but only imagined. The halos might be called the connecting link between imagination and sight. To see the halos is to improve the imagination, and the vision for the letters is also improved.

People with imperfect sight may also see the halos, though less perfectly, and when they understand that they are imagined, they often become able to imagine them where they had not been seen before, or to increase their vividness, in which case the sight always improves.

This can be done by imagining the appearances first with the eyes closed; and then looking at the card, or at fine print, and imagining them there. By alternating these two acts of imagination the sight is often improved rapidly.

One can improve the vision for reading not by looking at the letters, but by improving the imagination of the halos. To look at the letters very soon brings on a strain, with imperfect sight.

To look at the white spaces and to improve their whiteness, is a benefit to the imagination and to the vision. One cannot read fine print at all unless the halos are imagined.

It is best to begin the practice at the point at which the halos are seen, or can be imagined best. Nearsighted people are usually able to see them at the near-point, sometimes very vividly. Farsighted people may also see them best at this point, although their sight for form may be best at the distance.

By practice one becomes able to imagine or to see the halos more perfectly — the better the imagination, the better the sight.[49]

**Step 7 Summary – Holy Halos!**

- ✓ To reduce visual effort, see or imagine white spaces in and around black letters as brightly white.
- ✓ Use your memory and imagination of any bright white surface to increase the appearance of halos.

# Step 8. Guidance from a Bright White Line

[12] As you get used to imagining the white halos around letters and your ability to do so improves, you may also start to notice these halos blend together to form a bright white ribbon on which the black letters seem to rest. You may also see a thin bright white line underneath each line of text. This very thin line is bright, clear and distinct. It touches the bottom of the black letters and extends along the entire line of text. **The thinner this white line is imagined to be, the brighter it becomes.**

[11] The thin white line looks similar to the bright white line that appears at the very edge of a white piece of paper when it is placed near a light and held against another white paper.

When you see or imagine the thin bright white line, let your eyes shift easily and rapidly along it. Blink regularly and allow your head to freely move along. Of course, the eyes will shift from the thin white line to the letters in order to see them best. When your attention stays mainly with the thin white line, this shifting in and out of the letters is done so swiftly that you may not even notice doing it. Due to this unconscious rapid shifting, reading becomes a lot easier; the eyes relax further and vision improves for most people.

If you do not see the thin white line yet, close your eyes and imagine holding a fine paintbrush. Dip it in a pot of bright white paint and draw a thin white line beneath an imagined line of text. Notice how brightly the white paint contrasts with the black ink as you pull the brush along the line. Then open your eyes briefly and imagine drawing your white paintbrush underneath lines on this page.

Alternate imagining the thin white line with your eyes closed and glancing at it with your eyes open.

If it is hard to imagine a paintbrush, trace the thin white line with a pointer and let your eyes follow along. Use a pointer like the high-tech, no-expense-spared reading tool shown here, also known as a folded-out paperclip... The tip of a pencil will work equally well, or, if pointy tools are scarce, go ahead and use your index finger. Children do this too, because it works!

Move slowly at first; let your eyes get used to following the pointer. As you gradually increase speed you may notice the text slide across smoothly in the opposite direction.

Make no effort to either look at the black letters or at the white spaces. Your attention will inevitably shift to the letters on a regular basis. Always come back to the white line, and keep relaxing as you follow it along.

Hold this page at your optimal reading distance and practice tracing the thin white line in this text:

## The Thin White Line

by William H. Bates, M.D.

[13] When reading small print in a newspaper or in a book the normal eye is able to imagine the white spaces between the lines whiter than they really are. The whiter the spaces are imagined the blacker the letters appear and the more distinct do they become.

[12] Persons with imperfect sight do not become able to read fine print until they become able to imagine the white spaces between the lines of letters to be whiter than they really are.

[11] If one can imagine a thin white line below letters of the test card or beneath a line of fine print it is very helpful. This thin white line is only imagined, it is not seen, because the line is not really there. It is valuable in the treatment and cure of presbyopia, hypermetropia, astigmatism and many cases of myopia. It is well to imagine it in the right way. The wrong way is to try to imagine the thin white line and the black letters at the same time. This is a strain which always blurs the black letters and prevents the thin white line from being imagined.

[10] Many patients complain that they have difficulty in imagining the thin white line. To overcome this, one should imagine it just below some word or collection of words which are known. The line is then readily imagined and it can be imagined extending from one side of the page to the other, and wherever it becomes manifest the vision is always improved. One can read rapidly, clearly, and without discomfort, when he is conscious of the thin white line.

When the eyes look directly at the letters, an effort is required, while looking at the white spaces between the lines is a rest, and by practice in this way, one can become able to see the letters clearly, without looking directly at them. When a patient looks at the white spaces between the lines of ordinary book type, he can read for hours and no fatigue, pain or discomfort is felt. When discomfort and pain in the eyes is felt while reading, it is because the patient is looking directly at the letters.[50]

[12] It is sufficient to imagine the thin white line at the bottom of the letters. If you can imagine a thin white line at the top of the letters as easily as you imagine it at the bottom, feel free to do so.

Gradually hold text closer and continue to trace the thin white line in the most relaxed way; blink softly, breathe easily, shift your attention smoothly and continuously, allow your head to follow, and notice the letters, words, and page swinging. Rest your eyes often: close them for a while or look away into the distance.

You will remember from step 5 that it really helps to move the page side to side with a short smooth motion or that a slight side to side head motion increases relaxation and improves vision. Use such head or page motion while you follow the white lines, as this encourages eye motion. The only disadvantage of either side to side head or page motion is that there may be a tendency to stop and stare at the point of changing direction. You can avoid this with a two-dimensional swing, which creates continuous motion.

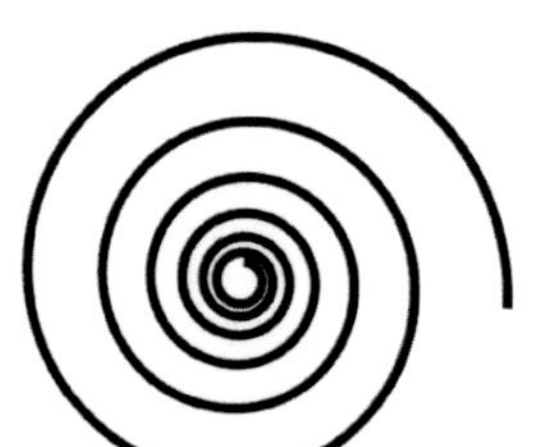

A gradually decreasing spiral that ends in a small circular swing is useful for general items you look at, whereas for reading a square swing with rounded edges is more suitable.

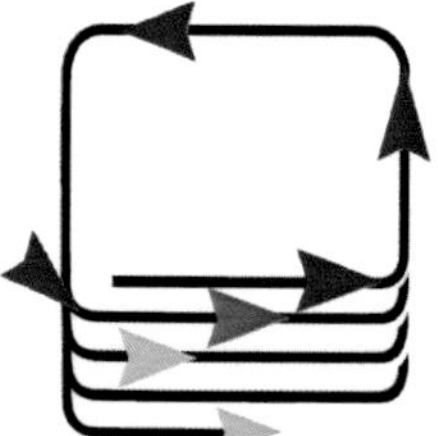

To use the square swing for reading: follow the thin white line underneath a line of text, then shift upward along the right margin to the top of the paragraph or page, where you shift back to the left and down to the next white line underneath text you want to read. When done smoothly, continuously and rapidly, this is an effective way of clearing the print and increasing your ease of reading.

What happens to letters when you choose not to read them and you just imagine painting white lines?

For most people, text clears right up and becomes easy to read. The clarity stays as long as your attention stays predominantly with the white line. If you switch to reading the black letters, they may quickly blur again.

Dr. Bates explains why this happens:

There are a number of causes of failure to read fine print. The most common problem is to look at the black letters and to pay no attention to the white spaces between the lines. Regarding the black letters always lowers the vision and requires an effort, a strain which the patient can always realize. Sometimes, the white spaces may be improved sufficiently so that one begins to read the fine print, and almost immediately the vision is lost because of the great temptation to look at the letters.

The thin, white line has been observed by many people who failed to read. In all cases, the white line was forgotten and an effort was made to read by looking at the letters. It seems to be a reaction of the human mind while using the eyes properly for people to at once stop using their eyes properly when their vision improves. They seem to think that they get a glimpse of good vision by the memory of the thin, white line, and all that they need is a start and that they can then get along without the thin white line. It is the thin white line that helps people to read and although I may caution them about looking at the letters, and have them demonstrate immediately that looking at the letters is a bad thing, they find it exceedingly difficult to confine their attention to it.

Over and over again, I have had them prove that testing the sight causes a strain which always lowers the vision. Testing the imagination is different and is less apt to cause a strain. A patient with presbyopia can look up at the ceiling or a white cloud in the sky, and remember or imagine a mental picture of a perfect white color, and do it without any conscious strain or effort. Just as soon as they look at the fine print, they forget their imagination and fail by making an effort to see.

One can read rapidly, clearly, and without discomfort, when he is conscious of the thin white line, but to fix the black letters and expect to read them is a mistake which very few teachers or students have observed. The fact that one cannot read properly when looking at the black letters should be more widely known.[51]

Do you recognize any of the above causes of failure to read small print?

Looking directly at the black letters, forgetting to use the white spaces and the thin white line, or testing your vision on small print are habits that increase visual strain rather than lessen it.

An additional disadvantage of looking directly at black letters is that you may read with a jumping or skipping motion from word to word; your eyes will de-focus as they jump and need to re-focus with each landing. And if you stare at each individual letter, your reading will be slow and strenuous. These are not the most relaxing ways to read. The solution is to keep your attention with the thin white line and the halos.

Every time you read, look for the white halos first. Relax further through imagining a thin bright white line. As your ability to imagine the thin white line improves, the black letters appear clearer. Do not rush to read those letters! Continue to enjoy the easy rhythm of tracing the white line.

**Dodge the print – Trust the process – Reap the rewards.**

[13] Practice tracing the thin white line on gradually smaller print. Use a pointer to help you. Blink softly, breathe easily, and relax even as the print gets smaller. Make no effort to read. The aim is to notice the white line and to see the print slide by smoothly as you trace the line.

> [12] Some time ago there was printed in this magazine a description of a method of curing astigmatism which is far superior to all other methods.
>
> [11] The patient was advised that there were white spaces between the lines of black letters and that these white spaces became whiter by alternately imagining them as white as possible with the eyes closed and then with the eyes open.
>
> [10] The attention of the patient was called to the fact that one could imagine the bottoms of the letters resting upon the upper part of the white spaces, and when the letters were read a thin white line could be imagined going across the card from left to right.
>
> [9] This thin white line was improved by the imagination of the line with the eyes alternately open and closed. When the imagination was successful in improving the thin white line, the black letters were imagined blacker and could usually be distinguished very quickly; but when the imagination of the white spaces was less perfect, the black letters could not usually be normally seen.
>
> [8] In other words, the improvement in the vision for the black letters depended primarily upon the improvement of the whiteness of the thin white line. Of the two the thin white line was more important because one can imagine the whiteness of the thin white line much whiter relatively than the imagination can picture the blackness of the black letters.[52]
>
> William H. Bates, M.D.

[12] **A Note on Speed Reading**

I am often asked whether speed reading courses are good for the eyes. So far I have never felt the need to take such a course, so I do not speak from personal experience, but I have been given examples by my students. My general impression of these courses is that they teach you to take in a whole paragraph or even a whole page at one glance. This can lead to conscious or subconscious diffusion of the eyes, which is a major strain and may lead to headaches as well as visual problems. Nearly all of my students who have tried speed-reading tell me it gives them a headache. If you experience problems while you speed-read, you are probably straining your eyes!

Dr. Bates did not recommend such strained methods of rapid reading and explains his thoughts:

> In my writings I have remonstrated against the methods employed to teach rapid reading. The usual procedure was to encourage the student to see all of the letters of a word at once, or to see all the letters of a paragraph of words at the same time. This was accepted as the correct method and very intelligent scholars have recommended it. My research work has proved that there is nothing more injurious to the eyes than to make an effort to see a whole letter or a whole word, all parts equally well. If one looks at the first letter of a word, the last letter is not seen perfectly at the same time. If an effort is made, the whole word becomes blurred and may not be distinguished. The stronger the effort that is made, the more injurious it is to the mind and eyes.[53]

My own experience is that I can read quite rapidly when I use my eyes the way Dr. Bates suggests; scanning over the white spaces in the text. This keeps the eyes moving swiftly and easily, there is no effort, and there is no conscious thought about my eyes. It is this ease of reading that allows for fast reading.

**Step 8 Summary – Guidance from a Bright White Line**

✓ Halos blend together to form a thin, bright white line underneath words and sentences.

✓ Tracing the thin white line, either mentally or with a pointer, encourages smooth, continuous eye motion and relaxed rapid reading.

# Step 9. Love the Fine Print

| Schoolbook Recommendations | |
|---|---|
| Age | Font size |
| 7 | 30 point |
| 7 | 24 point |
| 8 | 18 point |
| 8-9 | 14 point |
| 9-12 | 12 point |
| 12+ | 10 point |

[11] A general belief is that small print is bad for the eyes. In Dr. Bates' time, the British Association for the Advancement of Science published regulations that forbade the use of small print in schools for children under twelve. Reading was not allowed at all until age seven, and at that age only 24 and 30 point print would be permitted. This was gradually reduced until age twelve when regular size print was allowed. These measures were aimed at reducing myopia (near-sight) in school children.

Bates realized that large print is more of a strain on the eyes than small print, and his research showed that a strain to see at the near point always produces hyperopia (also known as hypermetropia, or far-sight). Hyperopia is so common in children that it is presumed to be the normal state of the immature eye and cannot be prevented. Eye doctors usually tell you that your child will grow out of it as their eyes grow.

Considering that large print actually contributes to the prevalence of hyperopia, it is no wonder hyperopia is so common among school children, and that the percentage tends to decline as they get older. Bates helped these children by giving them fine print to read and showed them how to overcome eyestrain. They were usually cured within a few visits. Adults had similar results.

> [10] **It is impossible to read fine print without relaxing. Therefore the reading of such print, contrary to what is generally believed, is a great benefit to the eyes.**[54]
>
> William H. Bates, M.D.

[11] The problem with large print is that it can still be read even when the eyes stare and diffuse, taking in a large area all at once. If you tend to strain to read, you can get away with it when reading large letters, but not with small. Any strain will quickly blur small print beyond the level of readability.

Small print requires focus on a small area. Just looking at fine print improves your level of central fixation – you make excellent use of your central clarity when you read it. You have to see your central point best in order to read small letters clearly. In addition, small print requires continual shifting, which relaxes your eyes.

[11] Prove it to yourself – look at this example:

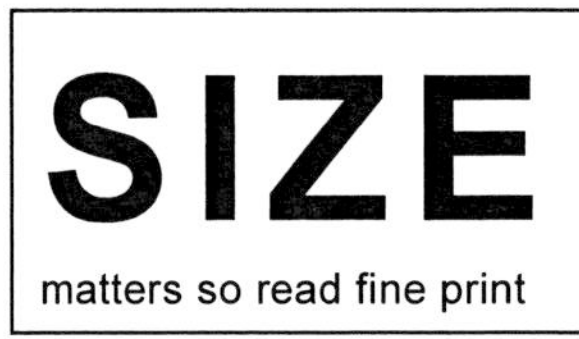


Look at the S in “SIZE”’ and check if you recognize the E in your peripheral vision while you look at the S. It is probably fairly easy to distinguish the E, correct?

Now look at the m in “matters” and check if at the same time you can also recognize the last letter on that line in your peripheral vision. This will be a challenge! And it should be.

You can read the whole word “SIZE” while you stare at the S, but to recognize all of the small print your eyes must shift along that line, even though the distance between the first and last letters is similar.

In essence: **reading small print requires smooth, continuous eye motion and relaxation.** This fact makes small print an excellent form of biofeedback – its degree of clarity or blurriness reflects your level of visual relaxation in that moment. Simply looking at fine print is a great way to practice and achieve relaxation.

Relax and blink as you read the following line down from 13 point font at the top to 4 point font at the bottom:

Look at small print for five minutes every day to help you regain central clarity.

Look at small print for five minutes every day to help you regain central clarity.

Look at small print for five minutes every day to help you regain central clarity.

Look at small print for five minutes every day to help you regain central clarity.

Look at small print for five minutes every day to help you regain central clarity.

Look at small print for five minutes every day to help you regain central clarity.

Look at small print for five minutes every day to help you regain central clarity.

Look at small print for five minutes every day to help you regain central clarity.

Look at small print for five minutes every day to help you regain central clarity.

Look at small print for five minutes every day to help you regain central clarity.

[11] A nice variation is to read the first word of each line from top to bottom, then the next word from bottom to top, and so on. Stay aware of the halos and notice how far down you can still make out each word without effort.

> Pam (age fifty-three):
> "It is pretty magical to read your text that decreases line by line. Overall I look at it and think this looks impossible but my eyes follow the words legibly to the end and voila I have been able to discern it all!"

Now practice your new reading skills on this small print:[55]

[6] Seven Truths of Normal Sight

1—Normal Sight can always be demonstrated in the normal eye, but only under favorable conditions.

2—Central Fixation: The letter or part of the letter regarded is always seen best.

3—Shifting: The point regarded changes rapidly and continuously.

4—Swinging: When the shifting is slow, the letters appear to move from side to side, or in other directions, with a pendulum-like motion.

5—Memory is perfect. The color and background of the letters, or other objects seen, are remembered perfectly, instantaneously and continuously.

6—Imagination is good. One may even see the white part of letters whiter than it really is, while the black is not altered by distance, illumination, size, or form, of the letters.

7—Rest or relaxation of the eye and mind is perfect and can always be demonstrated.

When one of these seven fundamentals is perfect, all are perfect.

## [12] **Can't read it yet? – Tips that may help**

- Hold small print at a distance where you see it best. Use the guidance from the previous steps to help clear the print. Remember to blink once or twice per line. Blinking regularly and softly is something that will become habitual, although at first you may consciously have to think about it. Your goal is to keep your eyes relaxed. You will want to practice reading this print with utmost ease!

- With small print, the halos are so close together that the thin white line becomes even more obvious. Your continuous awareness of the thin bright white line underneath the small print will let your eyes relax more and the print may start to clear.

- When the blur goes away, dodge any tendency to read the text. Avoid the temptation to try clear all the words. Keep blinking easily and frequently and continue to shift your attention along the white lines.

- Notice or imagine the apparent motion of letters and of the page as your eyes and head move smoothly along all the white spaces. This requires a relaxed awareness of peripheral vision.

- You may also benefit from briefly observing the blackness of the letters, and remembering this blackness with eyes alternately open and closed.

- When you hold text within your blur zone, reduce any tendency to stare by continuing to read at your normal speed as much as possible. For words that are not easily distinguished let your attention swing back and forth on the white underneath and between the letters.

- If small print is too blurry for you to read right now, it is beneficial to look at it without trying to read it. This will already help your vision; you learn to observe and notice smaller details.

## Step 9 Summary – Love the Fine Print

✓ Large print can be read with strain while small print requires relaxation.

✓ To keep or regain the ability to read small print close-up requires regularly looking at small print close-up.

# Step 10. Read Disclaimers by Candlelight

[12] Now that you have come this far, it is time to leave "Easy Street" and gradually change from reading under your most favorable conditions to reading under unfavorable conditions. As you know, disclaimers tend to be written in the smallest print so people are less likely to read them, and candlelight is considered insufficient light to read by, so reading disclaimers by candlelight may be the ultimate act of visual relaxation!

> [10] **Since small objects cannot be seen without central fixation, the reading of fine print, when it can be done, is one of the best of visual exercises, and the dimmer the light in which it can be read and the closer to the eye it can be held the better.**[56]
> William H. Bates, M.D.

Yes, despite what your mother may have told you, reading in bed by a dim light is good for your eyes, ***if*** you do it without effort. If you can read in a relaxed way under those difficult conditions, it will be even easier under favorable conditions. This applies equally to children and to adults. When you can stay relaxed and consciously avoid any temptation to strain to see under unfavorable conditions, your ability to read under favorable conditions will improve tremendously.

For people with presbyopia, unfavorable reading conditions typically are:

- smaller print,
- held closer to the eyes,
- in lower light, and
- with less contrast.

When you successfully master the first two – smaller print held closer to the eyes – the other two conditions will become less daunting too. You will soon read fancy menus printed on colored paper by candlelight!

[11] Bates used 'diamond' as his standard of small print.[57] His "Specimen of Diamond Type" printed on page 195 of *Perfect Sight Without Glasses* is approximately equivalent to 5 point in this book's times new roman font. In other fonts the point size can be slightly different.

| Times New Roman<br>5 point font: | Bookman Old Style<br>4.5 point font: |
|---|---|
| Dr. Bates recommended holding text of diamond size very close, at 6 inches or less from the eyes, even if you can't read the letters. When you do that, make no effort to read the text. Instead, close your eyes for a minute or two, and alternate that with looking at the small print for only a second or two. Imagine that the white background is perfectly white, and the letters are printed perfectly black. Can you improve on your imagination both with your eyes closed and with your eyes open? Simply observe what happens, and enjoy your path to clarity! | Dr. Bates recommended holding text of diamond size very close, at 6 inches or less from the eyes, even if you can't read the letters. When you do that, make no effort to read the text. Instead, close your eyes for a minute or two, and alternate that with looking at the small print for only a second or two. Imagine that the white background is perfectly white, and the letters are printed perfectly black. Can you improve on your imagination both with your eyes closed and with your eyes open? Simply observe what happens, and enjoy your path to clarity! |

I will describe four ways to improve your ability to read diamond print. Use each of these four suggestions with the diamond print practice cards provided on pages 137 and 139 and do most of what works best for you.

**1. Keep the eyes relaxed**

You may find it easiest to become comfortable with diamond print when you hold it at arm's length and, while looking at it, you make no effort to read it. To keep your eye muscles relaxed, I encourage you to give your eyes lots of rest. Much more than you think you need! So close your eyes until they feel so at ease that you hardly notice you have them. This may take a few minutes, but it may also take half an hour or longer, depending on your level of strain.

Then look at white spaces on the card with diamond print for just a few seconds. Close your eyes after those few seconds and deepen your level of relaxation. Alternate this rest with closed eyes with a few seconds of looking at the small print. You will likely find the print starts to clear up and may even become readable.

At first you may see the letters clearly only in brief flashes. That is great; it proves your eyes are capable of correct near focus! Keep going; you will soon see the letters clearly for longer, until finally you will be able to read them and retain the clarity. With continued practice you can reduce the distance until you read it at six inches.

**2. Attempt 'the impossible'**

Bring diamond print so close, four inches or less from your eyes, that you know for sure it is impossible to read. You can even let the paper touch your forehead and nose, and look directly at it without trying to read. Instant relaxation can sometimes be achieved when you believe there is absolutely no chance of reading it, because at that point you will not even try. As you give up on the mental effort, physical relaxation of your eyes follows.

While you hold the card with diamond print close to your eyes, accept any blur. Make no effort whatsoever to read the text. Either bring your attention to the white spaces and let your eyes glide smoothly across the page, or think of watching a football game, a ballet dancer, or flowers in your garden; whatever relaxes you! Continue until you can feel your eyes gradually relax, and wait for them to let go even further.

If you like, move the card slowly from side to side, about quarter of an inch is fine. The shorter and the slower the movement, the better it is, as long as you perceive some motion.

Close your eyes whenever any strain is felt, and keep them closed until the strain dissolves. You may need to close your eyes often at first. This is to be expected if you have not looked at anything so close to your eyes for quite some time. While your eyes are closed, either imagine that you are still looking at the page near your eyes and that you see it easily, free from strain, or that you are enjoying that football game, the ballet, or your garden.

After relaxing this way for a while the text may become clearer; it morphs from vague blurred lines to distinct words. The letters will likely seem larger than you expected and reading them becomes possible. Yet if you turn your mind to reading, the text may blur again. The old strain habit quickly returns and ruins your relaxation. The lesson is obvious – perfect vision comes through relaxation while any conscious effort to read, any trying, results in blur.

For best results Dr. Bates recommended doing this ultra-near vision practice as long as possible, even for many hours every day. Some people prefer to practice this with one eye at a time and cover the other eye or close it. Vary the hand which holds the card to avoid fatigue. The amount of light is not important.[58]

Let small print become your friend and daily companion! Look at fine print close-up for at least five minutes every day. Simply observe what happens, and enjoy the process. This relaxation practice at close range will be a great aid in regaining the ability to read average-size print at a comfortable reading distance.

************************

Let small print become your friend and daily companion!

Let small print become your friend and daily companion!

************************

**3. Use your memory and imagination**

One woman rapidly became able to read diamond print through her memory of white. Dr. Bates describes how he helped her:

> I handed her a small card on which was printed some lines of diamond type. I asked her what she could see. She said: "I see a gray card with a lot of blurred gray letters. They all seem to look alike and there are no spaces between the words or the letters and not always between the lines."
>
> I said to her: "With your eyes closed, can you remember such a thing as a sunset, a red sun and different colored clouds?"
> She said: "Yes."
>
> "With your eyes still closed, can you remember or imagine a white cloud in the sky, dazzling white with sun shining on it?"
> She answered: "Yes."
>
> Then I gave her the following directions: "Close your eyes, keeping them closed until you can remember a white cloud in the sky, dazzling white with the sun shining on it, then open your eyes and glance at the fine print, still remembering your white cloud, but be sure and close your eyes before you have time to read any of the letters." I watched her do this for a few minutes and saw that she was following my directions properly, then I left her to practice by herself.

After about half an hour I returned and asked her how she was getting along. Her face was a little bit flushed and in an apologetic tone she said: "I tried to do just exactly what you told me to do, Doctor, and I am sorry to say that although I only looked at the card for a second at a time, in flashes, contrary to your instructions, I read every word on the card." Then I explained to her that of course at the first visit she was not expected to do what I asked her to do exactly, but, under the circumstances, I thought that she had done very well indeed.

I gave her some other fine print to practice with in the same way, but to hold it not more than six inches from her eyes. With her eyes closed she remembered the white cloud as before, keeping her eyes closed until her memory of the white cloud was perfect, and then she flashed the white spaces between the lines for a second.

I watched her for a while, and I said: "What is the trouble?"

"Nothing," she said. "I close my eyes and remember the white cloud. I also remember it very well with my eyes open. When I do I cannot help seeing the white spaces perfectly white and the black letters perfectly black, but I am sorry to say that I cannot avoid reading the letters."

Then I held out my hand to her and said: "Shake hands. I am very well pleased with you and this time I will forgive you for not avoiding reading the letters."[59]

Dr. Bates tried the same method on many of his other patients but seldom found one who succeeded as well as this lady. Still, this imagination of a dazzling white alternated with flashing of the white spaces is worth practicing. If you do not succeed – move on to one of the other methods.

**4. You thought diamond was small???**

Another effective method for reading diamond print is to compare it to print that is even smaller…

Bates used fine print that had been reduced in size even further by photography. The result is 'microscopic print'. Miniature Bibles (see Resources, page 117) have this tiny print. A good printer can produce readable 'microscopic' text by using font size 2.5 or smaller.[60]

The beauty of this microscopic print is that just looking at it narrows down your point of focus. The smaller your point of focus, the better you see. This is true for as long as you keep a relaxed awareness of your peripheral vision at the same time and you smoothly let your attention shift from one point to the next. Effortlessly looking at microscopic print, even if you cannot read it (yet), promotes a natural use of your eyes.

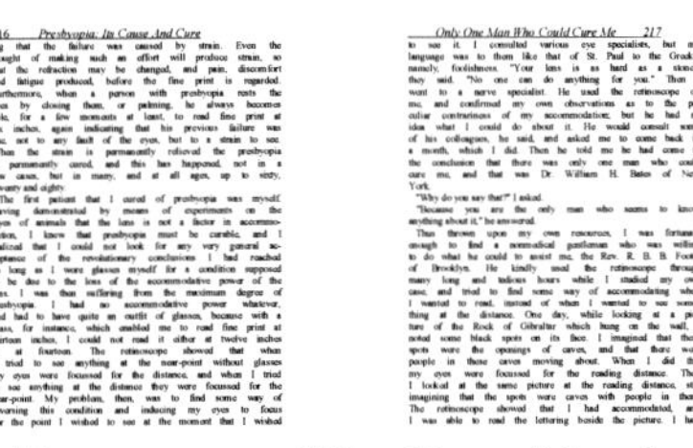

216 *Presbyopia: Its Cause And Cure*

ing that the failure was caused by strain. Even the thought of making such an effort will produce strain, so that the refraction may be changed, and pain, discomfort and fatigue produced, before the fine print is regarded. Furthermore, when a person with presbyopia rests the eyes by closing them, or palming, he always becomes able, for a few moments at least, to read fine print at six inches, again indicating that his previous failure was due, not to any fault of the eyes, but to a strain to see. When the strain is permanently relieved the presbyopia is permanently cured, and this has happened, not in a few cases, but in many, and at all ages, up to sixty, seventy and eighty.

The first patient that I cured of presbyopia was myself. Having demonstrated by means of experiments on the eyes of animals that the lens is not a factor in accommodation, I knew that presbyopia must be curable, and I realized that I could not look for any very general acceptance of the revolutionary conclusions I had reached so long as I wore glasses myself for a condition supposed to be due to the loss of the accommodative power of the lens. I was then suffering from the maximum degree of presbyopia. I had no accommodative power whatever, and had to have quite an outfit of glasses, because with a glass, for instance, which enabled me to read fine print at thirteen inches, I could not read it either at twelve inches or at fourteen. The retinoscope showed that when I tried to see anything at the near-point without glasses my eyes were focussed for the distance, and when I tried to see anything at the distance they were focussed for the near-point. My problem, then, was to find some way of reversing this condition and inducing my eyes to focus for the point I wished to see at the moment that I wished

*Only One Man Who Could Cure Me* 217

to see it. I consulted various eye specialists, but my language was to them like that of St. Paul to the Greeks, namely, foolishness. "Your lens is as hard as a stone," they said. "No one can do anything for you." Then I went to a nerve specialist. He used the retinoscope on me, and confirmed my own observations as to the peculiar contrariness of my accommodation; but he had no idea what I could do about it. He would consult some of his colleagues, he said, and asked me to come back in a month, which I did. Then he told me he had come to the conclusion that there was only one man who could cure me, and that was Dr. William H. Bates of New York.

"Why do you say that?" I asked.

"Because you are the only man who seems to know anything about it," he answered.

Thus thrown upon my own resources, I was fortunate enough to find a nonmedical gentleman who was willing to do what he could to assist me, the Rev. R. B. B. Foote, of Brooklyn. He kindly used the retinoscope through many long and tedious hours while I studied my own case, and tried to find some way of accommodating when I wanted to read, instead of when I wanted to see something at the distance. One day, while looking at a picture of the Rock of Gibraltar which hung on the wall, I noted some black spots on its face. I imagined that these spots were the openings of caves, and that there were people in these caves moving about. When I did this my eyes were focussed for the reading distance. Then I looked at the same picture at the reading distance, still imagining that the spots were caves with people in them. The retinoscope showed that I had accommodated, and I was able to read the lettering beside the picture. I had,

Two pages of Dr. Bates' book reduced to microscopic print.

The following practice will help you take advantage of this knowledge:

On page 135 you will find Dr. Bates' original "Fundamentals Card" followed by his "Seven Truths of Normal Sight" in diamond print on page 137. Underneath the diamond print you will see some microscopic print (font size 2). Hold these two pages at twelve inches from your eyes. Before you start, close your eyes for a while to let them rest.

When you open your eyes, look at the white margin of the page for no more than a second – a flash, similar to the photographs you took in step 2. With your eyes closed again remember the white you saw and imagine this white becoming brighter. Take another quick look at the white. Repeat this warm-up a few times.

Now proceed and look at the white spaces in the microscopic print for a second or two.
Then blink and similarly look at the white spaces in the diamond print.
Blink again and look at the white spaces in the lower lines of the Fundamentals card.
Blink again and shift up to a line you can read. Follow the thin white line underneath that line and then blink and shift back down to the microscopic print.

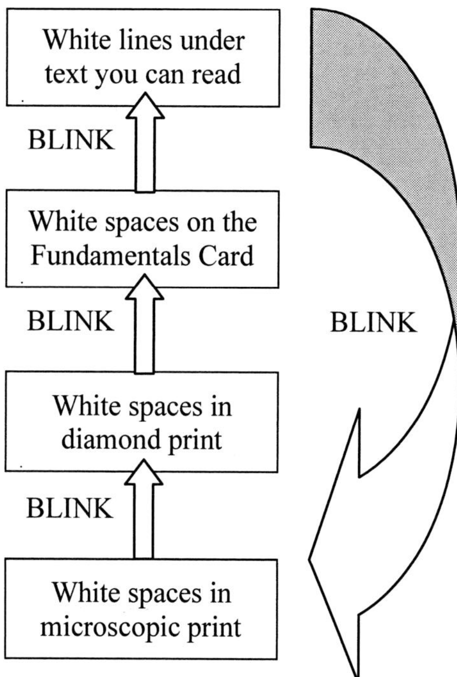


Repeat this until you can read all the lines of the Fundamental card and the diamond print.

Take your time! It will not happen in just a few minutes, but if you can stay relaxed with this, it is quite possible that you will read much better in twenty to thirty minutes or an hour. Regular daily practice will bring the best results. When the entire Fundamentals card becomes easy to read at twelve inches, move it closer, until you can read it at six inches or less.

If just blinking and shifting do not bring results for you, close your eyes longer between each shift and remember a bright white. When you open your eyes look for more white spaces, but only for a second, and then close your eyes again and repeat the process of remembering bright white before you flash the next white space.

**Looking at microscopic print leads to reading diamond print**

Dr. Bates and his assistant Emily Lierman (who later became his wife) often used microscopic print, and they described several cases to illustrate how they used it to improve reading ability in presbyopic patients. One of these patients was a man of sixty-four who used reading glasses for all text sizes. Emily writes:

> I have been treating a man, aged sixty-four, with presbyopia. The vision of both his eyes was the same, namely 15/30. He could not read newspaper nor magazine type at all without glasses. Closing his eyes often to rest them helped.
>
> I was anxious to help him to read fine print or diamond type. During one of his previous treatments, I helped him to read newspaper and magazine type, which was an encouragement to him. When the fine print was placed about eight inches from his eyes, he asked: "You don't think I will ever be able to read such fine type as that, do you?"
> This question amused me, because most patients with presbyopia ask the same question.
> I answered: "Yes, I know you will."
>
> With a great deal of doubt in his mind, he followed my advice. He was given a booklet, which contains microscopic print, and told to hold it about eight inches from his eyes. Then directly above this print was placed the small diamond type card, which describes the Seven Truths of Normal Sight. Then above this was placed another, a little larger in size, describing the fundamentals of treatment by W. H. Bates, M.D. This card is made up of different sized type, which starts rather large at the top and graduates down to fine reading type at the very bottom of the card.
>
> The patient was directed to look at the white spaces between the microscopic type; then blink and shift his eyes to the white spaces of the diamond type; then blink and shift again to the larger white spaces of the Fundamental card. In this way, my patient read sentence after sentence of the Fundamentals until he had read the very small print at the bottom of the card. The patient is grateful for learning how to use his eyes normally.[61]

A similar case was a lady of sixty-three, who had worn glasses for more than thirty years and during the past two years her eye specialist found it difficult to fit her with glasses correctly. She had purchased her last pair the day before she came to Dr. Bates' office, and told Emily those glasses made her so nervous and irritable that she could not possibly wear them more than half a day. Her distance vision was normal but when she held the Fundamentals card at arm's length she said that she knew there was some kind of print on the card but could not tell what it was. In despair she looked at Emily and said, "I fear you will have a hard time getting me to read this."

Emily told her to look at the small white spaces between the lines of print in the microscopic type, close both eyes and remember the white spaces. She could remember them white with her eyes closed. She was then told to open her eyes and again look at the white spaces. She said they appeared whiter than they had the first time. Again Emily told her to close her eyes and remember the white spaces and to open them for less than a second, look at the white spaces of the diamond type card, close her eyes and remember the white spaces; then for just a second to open her eyes and look at the white spaces of the fundamental card.

The lady practiced this for almost a half hour, with the result that she could read the entire fundamental card at eight inches from her eyes. You will find the full story on page 114.

I used the same process with Gene, a man of sixty-one with 2.25 diopters of presbyopia and a similar level of astigmatism. In his first session I placed the large practice chart at six feet and helped him relax his eyes before I let him move on to the medium chart held at arm's length. When I handed him the Better Eyesight card (page 141) he blurted:
"Forget that; I can barely read the top two paragraphs!"

Instead of returning to the easy larger charts I told him to hold the card with diamond and microscopic print (page 137) at the bottom of the Better Eyesight card. I instructed him to look at the white spaces in the microscopic print first, then to blink and work his way up to those top paragraphs. Despite doubting my sanity he followed my instructions and within ten minutes he was happily reading font size 8, paragraph 9 on the card.

**Step 10 Summary – Read Disclaimers by Candlelight**

- ✓ When you have regained the ability to read regular print at a comfortable reading distance it is time to practice with even smaller print closer to your eyes.
- ✓ Diamond and microscopic print are excellent practice fonts!
- ✓ Alternate looking at microscopic, diamond and regular print with ease and regular soft blinking.
- ✓ Continue to improve your near vision: gradually decrease the amount of light and practice with text on colored backgrounds.

# Throw Away Your Reading Glasses!

[11] Daily practice of the ten steps to reading without glasses creates steady progress on your path to clear vision. Although you may practice one step at a time, in the process of natural vision all the relaxed vision habits are to a great extent interdependent. Healthy eyes continually move, blink and see with central clarity while noticing peripheral motion. They are light-finders; they love contrast and imaginary halos and they can pick up the smallest detail and the slightest change in hue. They never strain to see, regardless of conditions.

Such happy eyes follow the mind's attention – swiftly, effortlessly and accurately – regardless of distance. When you keep this in mind and replace any acquired strained vision habits with the natural ways of seeing, your eyes will serve you well for the rest of your life.

**It is the things that we stop doing that promote the memory of perfect sight. We do not need to practice something new nor learn by mental training how to do something that we have never done before. When a patient is convinced of these facts [he realizes that] using his eyes correctly is so much easier and brings renewed vision.**[62]

William H. Bates, M.D.

**Your investment**

The more time you spend looking at details at the near point, without strain or glasses of course, the sooner your eyes regain their ability to focus at close range. Even five minutes of daily relaxation practice can bring amazing results. When you practice more than five minutes per day you will reap rewards sooner. When you relax how you see all day long, at all distances, your improvement will be most rapid, and lasting clear vision will be your reward.

**Improve and maintain clarity**

If you used lower diopter glasses to read this book, these glasses will soon give a vision acuity as clear as your regular glasses provided. When that happens it is time to drop another quarter diopter or more and repeat the process until you can easily read without glasses.

To maintain clarity all that is required is to keep using your eyes in this relaxed way. A daily habit of reading small print at the near point with all the correct vision habits ensures you will avoid the need for reading glasses at any age.

[8] You will love the joy of reading tiny print again at any distance.

[6] Let me know when you get to that point!!!

**The 10 steps in review:**

Step 1. **Become aware of eyestrain** and other factors that contribute to blurry vision, so you can begin to turn the tide. Stop using reading glasses or temporarily use lower-strength glasses or pinhole glasses. Accept your blurry vision; never strain to see.

Step 2. **Rest your eyes** with palming, sunning and massage. Close your eyes whenever they feel tired and keep them closed until they feel rested. Blink regularly and easily. Good posture helps to release eye muscle tension. Imagine clarity at the near point. Let images of achieving your goal of excellent vision inspire you!

Step 3. Once your eyes are rested, begin with **your most favorable conditions** in terms of light, print size, and distance. Choose inspiring texts and aim for optimal nutrition.

Step 4. **Practice seeing effortlessly at the near point** with some near-vision warm-ups using the palm of your hand or fun, colorful objects. Enjoy close encounters. Make good use of your memory and imagination.

Step 5. **Move** your head or the page and relax your neck and eye muscles through motion. Swing side to side, as well as back and forth in and out of your blur zone to invite the eyes to focus. Notice apparent motion all day long.

Step 6. **Improve your central clarity.** Practice seeing one letter best at a time, then part of a letter better than the rest of the same letter. Progress gradually from large to small print and from far to near. Avoid the tunnel vision trap with a relaxed awareness of your entire field of vision.

Step 7. When you let your eyes be the light-finders they are, you can imagine the white in and around letters to be brighter white and you will **notice halos** that make the black letters stand out darker. Here too, gradually progress from large letters to small, and use your memory and imagination.

Step 8. **Follow the thin bright white line** underneath lines of text. Let it effortlessly guide your attention along the bottom of the print. When you keep your attention mostly with the thin bright white line, reading becomes effortless. Practice with text at your optimal distances for fastest improvement.

Step 9. **Love the fine print!** Small print stimulates natural correct use of the eyes, as long as you do not strain to read it. Begin at your optimal distance and read at your normal speed as much as possible. Gradually decrease the distance at which you hold it.

Step 10. **Read disclaimers by candlelight** or at least practice relaxing with diamond print at four inches from your eyes. Make smart use of microscopic print and dim light. Let your imagination clear the print, even if it seems impossible to read. Oh, and throw away those glasses…

**Focus challenges**

Sometimes in life you get thrown in the deep end before you have learned to swim with confidence. If that happens, don't worry! On occasions where light and print size are not under your control and you are tempted to use your glasses, use the following 'quick fix' list instead. You may find the readers can stay in your pocket.

**QUICK FIX READING**

| | DOs | DON'Ts |
|---|---|---|
| 1. | DO accept any blur. | DON'T squint, strain or fight the blur. |
| 2. | DO blink regularly and close your eyes to rest them as needed. | DON'T keep tired eyes open. |
| 3. | DO open your peripheral vision. | DON'T narrow down to tunnel vision. |
| 4. | DO notice white spaces or background on the page. | DON'T make an effort to see or to read the letters. |
| 5. | DO shift your attention smoothly and continuously. (Slight page and/or head motion will help a lot!) | DON'T stare at the letters or at any point. |
| 6. | DO focus your mind. Be interested in the page. | DON'T attempt to focus your eyes. |
| 7. | DO imagine halos and the thin white line. | DON'T try to see blacker letters. |
| 8. | DO remember the letters are printed clearly with black ink. Imagine you already see them clearly. | DON'T think the text is printed in gray blur. |

[12] **Differences in visual habits**

There are distinct differences in how people with clear vision use their eyes compared to those who have blurred vision. The latter group can copy the habits of the former group and use their healthy habits as a guide to clear vision. Here is an overview of the differences:

| People with clear vision | People with blurred near vision |
|---|---|
| generally relax to see better. | generally strain to see better. |
| see best with central vision. | may see best with peripheral vision. |
| are aware of their whole peripheral field. | tend to fall into tunnel vision mode. |
| blink regularly and easily. | blink rarely and/or with effort. |
| shift smoothly, rapidly, with small saccades (natural involuntary movements) of 60 to 100 times per second. | shift slowly or haltingly, with a tendency to stop and stare. |
| let the head follow the eyes smoothly. | hold the head still while the eyes move. |
| read smoothly and rapidly. More attention is given to the white spaces than to black print (albeit often subconsciously). | read slowly and haltingly; an effort is made to see the black print. |
| see or imagine spaces in and around letters to be bright white. | see or imagine spaces in and around letters to be gray. |
| see black letters perfectly black. Letter size and form is perceived accurately. | may see black letters as gray, with blurred edges, or with multiple images. Letter size appears smaller than reality. |
| notice objects move with a gentle continuous swing. | observe objects as stationary or with an irregular swing. |
| see a field of perfect black while palming. | see a field of gray and black mixed with colors and moving lights while palming. |
| are comfortable in bright sunlight without sunglasses. | squint or use sunglasses in bright sunlight. |

# Inspirational Stories

[12] You may be inspired to throw away your reading glasses even sooner by reading about people who overcame their presbyopia using the Bates Method.

One delightful example comes from my colleague Trudy Eyges who teaches the Bates Method in Massachusetts. She has been on the faculties of Cornell, Wellesley and MIT teaching French and English. After she retired in her sixties she read Aldous Huxley's book *The Art of Seeing* which introduced her to the Bates Method. She decided, out of sheer curiosity, to test the method for herself and began a daily practice of visual relaxation techniques.

After two short weeks of practicing she chucked her glasses that she had been wearing for forty years! That day she picked up a paper from her kitchen table and read it. She finished reading and then realized her glasses were not on her nose, yet she had just read this paper with ease and clarity. Her renewed ability to read without glasses surprised her, and she admits it was a bit of a shock. She then bought all the books on the Bates Method she could find and started giving workshops on the method.

Today, at age 92, Trudy still reads without glasses and also drives with ease, even at night. She continues to practice the Bates Method for a few minutes every day to care for her own eyesight and she continues to teach others. Testimonies from her students are so compelling that Senator Brownsberger at the Boston State House has filed a bill to have an eye chart put in every classroom.

Trudy's advice is: "Expect healing! Expect clarity to happen, yet you cannot force anything. Whose eyes are more important than yours?!? With commitment and daily practice, you can preserve your sight."[63]

On the following pages you will find more inspirational and educational stories, in a range of print sizes (from 11 to 4 point font) for your relaxed reading practice.
The first and last of these stories are repeated a few times in progressively smaller print so you can check back with larger print when small print becomes challenging. In doing so you will reduce strain and may find that you can continue to relax and read the smaller print.

## Prevention of Presbyopia is Easy

by William H. Bates, M.D.

[11]

While it is sometimes very difficult to cure presbyopia, it is, fortunately, very easy to prevent it. Oliver Wendell Holmes told us how to do it in "The Autocrat of the Breakfast Table," and it is astonishing, not only, that no attention was paid to his advice, but that we should be warned against the very course which was found so beneficial in the case he records:

"There is now living in New York State," he says, "an old gentleman who, perceiving his sight to fail, immediately took to exercising it on the finest print, and in this way fairly bullied Nature out of her foolish habit of taking liberties at the age of forty-five or thereabouts. And now this old gentleman performs the most extraordinary feats with his pen, showing that his eyes must be a pair of microscopes. I should be afraid to say how much he writes in the compass of a half dime, whether the Psalms or the Gospels, or the Psalms and the Gospels, I won't be positive."

Persons whose sight is beginning to fail at the near-point, or who are approaching the presbyopic age should imitate the example of this remarkable old gentleman. Get a specimen of diamond type, and read it every day in an artificial light, bringing it closer and closer to the eye till it can be read at six inches or less. Or get a specimen of type reduced by photography until it is much smaller than diamond type, and do the same. You will thus escape, not only the necessity of wearing glasses for reading and near work, but all of those eye troubles which now so often darken the latter years of life.[64]

## Prevention of Presbyopia is Easy

by William H. Bates, M.D.

[8]

While it is sometimes very difficult to cure presbyopia, it is, fortunately, very easy to prevent it. Oliver Wendell Holmes told us how to do it in "The Autocrat of the Breakfast Table," and it is astonishing, not only, that no attention was paid to his advice, but that we should be warned against the very course which was found so beneficial in the case he records:

"There is now living in New York State," he says, "an old gentleman who, perceiving his sight to fail, immediately took to exercising it on the finest print, and in this way fairly bullied Nature out of her foolish habit of taking liberties at the age of forty-five or thereabouts. And now this old gentleman performs the most extraordinary feats with his pen, showing that his eyes must be a pair of microscopes. I should be afraid to say how much he writes in the compass of a half dime, whether the Psalms or the Gospels, or the Psalms and the Gospels, I won't be positive."

Persons whose sight is beginning to fail at the near-point, or who are approaching the presbyopic age should imitate the example of this remarkable old gentleman. Get a specimen of diamond type, and read it every day in an artificial light, bringing it closer and closer to the eye till it can be read at six inches or less. Or get a specimen of type reduced by photography until it is much smaller than diamond type, and do the same. You will thus escape, not only the necessity of wearing glasses for reading and near work, but all of those eye troubles which now so often darken the latter years of life.

# Prevention of Presbyopia is Easy

by William H. Bates, M.D.

[7]

While it is sometimes very difficult to cure presbyopia, it is, fortunately, very easy to prevent it. Oliver Wendell Holmes told us how to do it in "The Autocrat of the Breakfast Table," and it is astonishing, not only, that no attention was paid to his advice, but that we should be warned against the very course which was found so beneficial in the case he records:

"There is now living in New York State," he says, "an old gentleman who, perceiving his sight to fail, immediately took to exercising it on the finest print, and in this way fairly bullied Nature out of her foolish habit of taking liberties at the age of forty-five or thereabouts. And now this old gentleman performs the most extraordinary feats with his pen, showing that his eyes must be a pair of microscopes. I should be afraid to say how much he writes in the compass of a half dime, whether the Psalms or the Gospels, or the Psalms and the Gospels, I won't be positive."

Persons whose sight is beginning to fail at the near-point, or who are approaching the presbyopic age should imitate the example of this remarkable old gentleman. Get a specimen of diamond type, and read it every day in an artificial light, bringing it closer and closer to the eye till it can be read at six inches or less. Or get a specimen of type reduced by photography until it is much smaller than diamond type, and do the same. You will thus escape, not only the necessity of wearing glasses for reading and near work, but all of those eye troubles which now so often darken the latter years of life.


## Prevention of Presbyopia is Easy

by William H. Bates, M.D.


[5]


While it is sometimes very difficult to cure presbyopia, it is, fortunately, very easy to prevent it. Oliver Wendell Holmes told us how to do it in "The Autocrat of the Breakfast Table," and it is astonishing, not only, that no attention was paid to his advice, but that we should be warned against the very course which was found so beneficial in the case he records:

"There is now living in New York State," he says, "an old gentleman who, perceiving his sight to fail, immediately took to exercising it on the finest print, and in this way fairly bullied Nature out of her foolish habit of taking liberties at the age of forty-five or thereabouts. And now this old gentleman performs the most extraordinary feats with his pen, showing that his eyes must be a pair of microscopes. I should be afraid to say how much he writes in the compass of a half dime, whether the Psalms or the Gospels, or the Psalms and the Gospels, I won't be positive."

Persons whose sight is beginning to fail at the near-point, or who are approaching the presbyopic age should imitate the example of this remarkable old gentleman. Get a specimen of diamond type, and read it every day in an artificial light, bringing it closer and closer to the eye till it can be read at six inches or less. Or get a specimen of type reduced by photography until it is much smaller than diamond type, and do the same. You will thus escape, not only the necessity of wearing glasses for reading and near work, but all of those eye troubles which now so often darken the latter years of life.



## Prevention of Presbyopia is Easy

by William H. Bates, M.D.


[4]


While it is sometimes very difficult to cure presbyopia, it is, fortunately, very easy to prevent it. Oliver Wendell Holmes told us how to do it in "The Autocrat of the Breakfast Table," and it is astonishing, not only, that no attention was paid to his advice, but that we should be warned against the very course which was found so beneficial in the case he records:

"There is now living in New York State," he says, "an old gentleman who, perceiving his sight to fail, immediately took to exercising it on the finest print, and in this way fairly bullied Nature out of her foolish habit of taking liberties at the age of forty-five or thereabouts. And now this old gentleman performs the most extraordinary feats with his pen, showing that his eyes must be a pair of microscopes. I should be afraid to say how much he writes in the compass of a half dime, whether the Psalms or the Gospels, or the Psalms and the Gospels, I won't be positive."

Persons whose sight is beginning to fail at the near-point, or who are approaching the presbyopic age should imitate the example of this remarkable old gentleman. Get a specimen of diamond type, and read it every day in an artificial light, bringing it closer and closer to the eye till it can be read at six inches or less. Or get a specimen of type reduced by photography until it is much smaller than diamond type, and do the same. You will thus escape, not only the necessity of wearing glasses for reading and near work, but all of those eye troubles which now so often darken the latter years of life.

# Presbyopia, Its Cause and Cure

by William H. Bates, M.D.

[10]

The first patient that I cured of presbyopia was myself. Having demonstrated by means of experiments on the eyes of animals that the lens is not a factor in accommodation, I knew that presbyopia must be curable, and I realized that I could not look for any very general acceptance of the revolutionary conclusions I had reached so long as I wore glasses myself for a condition supposed to be due to the loss of the accommodative power of the lens. I was then suffering from the maximum degree of presbyopia.

I had no accommodative power whatever, and had to have quite an outfit of glasses, because with a glass, for instance, which enabled me to read fine print at thirteen inches, I could not read it either at twelve inches or at fourteen. The retinoscope showed that when I tried to see anything at the near-point without glasses my eyes were focused for the distance, and when I tried to see anything at the distance they were focused for the near-point.

My problem, then, was to find some way of reversing this condition and inducing my eyes to focus for the point I wished to see at the moment that I wished to see it. I consulted various eye specialists, but my language was to them like that of St. Paul to the Greeks, namely, foolishness. "Your lens is as hard as a stone," they said. "No one can do anything for you." Then I went to a nerve specialist. He used the retinoscope on me, and confirmed my own observations as to the peculiar contrariness of my accommodation; but he had no idea what I could do about it. He would consult some of his colleagues, he said, and asked me to come back in a month, which I did. Then he told me he had come to the conclusion that there was only one man who could cure me, and that was Dr. William H. Bates of New York.
"Why do you say that?" I asked.
"Because you are the only man who seems to know anything about it," he answered.

Thus thrown upon my own resources, I was fortunate enough to find a nonmedical gentleman who was willing to do what he could to assist me, the Rev. R. B. B. Foote, of Brooklyn. He kindly used the retinoscope through many long and tedious hours while I studied my own case, and tried to find some way of accommodating when I wanted to read, instead of when I wanted to see something at the distance. One day, while looking at a picture of the Rock of Gibraltar which hung on the wall, I noted some black spots on its face. I imagined that these spots were the openings of caves, and that there were people in these caves moving about. When I did this my eyes were focused for the reading distance. Then I looked at the same picture at the reading distance, still imagining that the spots were caves with people in them. The retinoscope showed that I had accommodated, and I was able to read the lettering beside the picture. I had, in fact, been temporarily cured by the use of my imagination. Later I found that when I imagined the letters black I was able to see them black, and when I saw them black I was able to distinguish their form.

My progress after this was not what could be called rapid. It was six months before I could read the newspapers with any kind of comfort, and a year before I obtained my present accommodative range of fourteen inches, from four inches to eighteen; but the experience was extremely valuable, for I had in pronounced form every symptom subsequently observed in other presbyopic patients.

Fortunately for the patients, it has seldom taken me as long to cure other people as it did to cure myself. In some cases a complete and permanent cure was effected in a few minutes. Why, I do not know. I will never be satisfied till I find out. A patient who had worn glasses for presbyopia for about twenty years was cured in less than fifteen minutes by the use of his imagination. When asked to read diamond type, he said he could not do so, because the letters were grey and looked all alike. I reminded him that the type was printer's ink and that there was nothing blacker than printer's ink. I asked him if he had ever seen printer's ink. He replied that he had. Did he remember how black it was? Yes. Did he believe that these letters were as black as the ink he remembered? He did, and then he read the letters; and because the improvement in his vision was permanent, he said that I had hypnotized him. In another case a presbyope of ten years' standing was cured just as quickly by the same method. When reminded that the letters which he could not read were black, he replied that he knew they were black, but that they looked grey.
"If you know they are black, and yet see them grey," I said, "you must imagine them grey. Suppose you imagine that they are black. Can you do that?"
"Yes," he said, "I can imagine that they are black"; and then he proceeded to read them.

These extremely quick cures are rare. In nine cases out of ten progress has been much slower, and it has been necessary to resort to all the methods of obtaining relaxation found useful in the treatment of other errors of refraction.[65]

## Effects of Presbyopia

by William H. Bates, M.D.

[10]

Patients who have been cured of presbyopia, which is caused by eyestrain, are able to do more satisfactory work than those who have imperfect sight and wear glasses. We receive many reports from patients who have had difficulties in their special line of work and have found that they accomplished more and were more accurate after their presbyopia was cured. Frequently, people of fifty years or more, lose their positions because of mistakes made in figures or whatever their work may be. They are not always told the reason for their dismissal. They are simply discharged and a younger man put in their place.

One of my patients, sixty-four years old, told me that, after having worked faithfully and steadily for forty years in one place, he had been informed that he could no longer figure accurately. It was a shock to him when he was placed on half pay and sent to another department. He was presbyopic, but was cured by treatment without glasses. During the absence of the younger man, he was temporarily placed in his former position. His work was so accurate and efficient that he was reinstated permanently.

Artists have the same experience with colors. It can be demonstrated that colors, when seen under a magnifying glass, become less distinct. White becomes a shade of gray; black becomes a lighter shade of black. It can also be shown that objects seen through glasses do not appear to be of the same size as the same objects viewed with the naked eye.

Many artists are disappointed with their work because for some good reason they feel that it is not appreciated. The great mistake they make is that, like other people suffering from presbyopia, they believe that because their ability to read is improved with glasses, their perception of colors and form is also benefited. It is not always easy to convince artists that glasses actually lower their vision not only for colors, but also for form.[66]

## Fine Print

by William H. Bates, M.D.

[10]

When people are able to read fine print with perfect sight at six inches or further, the white spaces between the lines are seen or imagined whiter than the rest of the card.

The ability to imagine the white spaces between the lines to be very white is accomplished by the memory of white snow, white starch or anything perfectly white, with the eyes closed for part of a minute. Some patients count thirty while remembering some white object or scene with the eyes closed. Then when the eyes are opened for a second, the white spaces between the lines of black letters are imagined or seen much whiter than before. By alternately remembering something perfectly white with the eyes closed and opening them for a few seconds and flashing the spaces, the vision or the imagination of the white spaces improves.

One needs to be careful not to make an effort or to regard the black letters. When the white spaces between the lines are imagined sufficiently white, or as white as they can be remembered with the eyes closed and with the eyes open, the black letters are read without effort or strain, or without the consciousness of regarding the black letters.

Many people discover that they can imagine a thin white line where the bottom of the letters comes in contact with the white spaces. This thin line is very white, and the thinner it is imagined to be, the whiter it becomes. When it is imagined perfectly, the letters are read without the consciousness of looking at them and the vision or imagination of the white is very much improved. This thin white line can be imagined much whiter than any other part of the page, and is more easily imagined or seen than any other part. Of course, the eyes have to shift from the thin, white line to the letters in order to see them, but the shifting is done so readily, so continuously, so perfectly that the reader does not notice that he is continually shifting. When the vision of the thin, white line is imperfect, the shifting is slow and imperfect and the vision for the letters is impaired.

The memory or the imagination of the thin, white line is usually so easy, so perfect and so continuous that everything regarded is seen with maximum vision. Patients with cataract who become able to imagine this thin, white line perfectly, very soon become able to read the finest print without effort or strain, and the cataract always improves, or becomes less. Patients with hypermetropia, astigmatism, squint, diseases of the retina and optic nerve are benefited in every way by the memory or the imagination of the thin, white line. Reading fine print with perfect sight benefits or improves all organic diseases of the eye.[67]

# Stories from the Clinic ~ Three Cases of Presbyopia

by Emily C. Lierman

[9]

As a rule more children than adults come to the clinic. They are sent to us by the schools, usually because they cannot see the blackboard. But during the war it was astonishing how many women came to us. Many of them were employed in factories where American flags were manufactured and could not see to do the work properly, although their sight at the distance seemed to be satisfactory. Some had trouble in threading their needles. Others complained that they saw double. One told me that she sometimes stitched her fingers to the blue field of the flag along with the Stars. They all asked for glasses, of course, but were very glad to learn that they could be cured so that they could see without them.

Among these very interesting patients was a woman of about fifty who had great trouble in threading her needle, and who begged me to help her because she had her living to earn. She spoke with a pronounced Irish accent, and was very amusing. Her distant vision was quickly improved by palming and flashing the letters on the Snellen test card. Then I suggested that she practice with fine print six inches from her eyes. Even though she did not see the letters, I told her, it would help her to alternately rest her eyes by closing for a few minutes and then look at the small letters for a couple of seconds. She got immediate results from this and was enthusiastic in her expressions of appreciation.

"Sure, ma'am, may the good angels bless you for that!" she exclaimed. "I think this very minute I would be threadin' a needle if I had one. Me old man and the young ones at home will think it foine to have meself threadin' a needle."

It seemed that members of her family had been called upon to thread her needles, and had found the task somewhat irksome.

The next clinic day she came again, and, although it was afternoon greeted me vociferously with the Irish salutation

"Top o' the mornin' to you!"

"Top o' the morning to yourself!" said I, and then I suggested that she should not speak so loud, as I was afraid she would disturb the other patients.

I am not sure that she did any harm, however. The patients all smiled at her remark, even the Jewish patients, who, I imagine, could not have understood it. It does me good to see these poor unfortunates smile a little, and I think it must do them good also.

She soon became able to thread her needle without any trouble, and she wanted everyone in the room to know it. The last time I saw her she said:

"Sure, ma'am, me eyes are very sharp now, for the minute I set eyes on me man when he comes home at night I can tell by the twinkle in his eye whether he has had anything stronger than water or tea."

Another woman, forty-eight years of age, told me that the first time she came to the clinic she thought she had got into the wrong place. Half a dozen people had their eyes covered with the palms of their hands, to rest them, and she thought it was a prayer meeting. It was she who sewed her fingers to the flag along with the Stars.

"What I need is glasses," she said, "and that's what I am here for"; but I soon convinced her that the glasses were unnecessary.

By having her alternately close and open her eyes I improved her sight for the Snellen test card from 15/40 to 15/20. Then I gave her some fine print to read, but it was only a blur to her. I now told her to palm, and imagine that she was sewing stars to the flag. When she opened her eyes her sight was worse. The very thought of those stars increased her strain and made her vision worse. This convinced her that her trouble was due to strain, and that all she needed was to get rid of the strain. I now asked her to imagine more agreeable objects at the near-point. She at once became able to read the fine print, and her sight for the distance also improved. After four visits to the clinic her vision both for the distance and the near-point had become almost normal. It was quite easy for her to thread a needle and to do her work without glasses.

A woman of seventy-four who has been coming to the clinic for some time works every day in an orphanage where she mends the children's clothes, and does other sewing. She complained that her glasses did not fit her, and she could no longer see to sew with them. I gave her a small card with some fine print on the back.
"Do you mean to tell me," she asked, "that I will ever read that?"
"It is possible." I said.

Her smiling face was good to see, as she tried to do as I instructed her. The print was larger on one side of the card than on the other, and I asked her to read the name printed in the larger letters. She could not do so at first. I told her to close her eyes, count ten, then open them and look at the card while she counted two, then repeat. In a few minutes she saw the name on the card and also the phone number. I had had her do the same thing with the diamond type on the reverse side, and after a while she became able to see some of the letters. At later visits she obtained further improvement, and after some months she had no difficulty in sewing the buttons on the children's clothes, without her glasses, although as she said, there were a lot of them and they kept her busy.[68]

## From an Old Man of Forty-Eight to a Young Man of Fifty

by E.F. Darling, M.D.

[10]

I have been practicing medicine as an ophthalmologist for the last twenty years. During a period of eighteen years prior to 1923, I spent a large part of my time putting glasses on my helpless patients. However, for the last two years I have been trying to make amends by removing their glasses as rapidly as possible.

I was wearing convex 2.25 D.S. for distance and convex 4.25 for reading. My distance vision had deteriorated in the eighteen years I had worn glasses, from better than normal to about one-third normal. My near vision had gone back so much that I was wearing the glass which theoretically should suit a person sixty or seventy years old. With the glasses off I could see only the largest headlines on the newspapers. While wearing the glasses, I had occasional headaches and eye aches, and my near vision was at times very defective, so that I had difficulty in doing fine work of any kind.

The first day I went around without glasses everything seemed blurred, but I felt somehow that I had gotten rid of some particularly galling chains. It was pleasant to feel the air blowing against my eyes, and I walked around the whole afternoon trying to get used to the new condition.

In carrying out the suggestions in Dr. Bates' book, I had a great deal of trouble for the first week or so, especially with the mental images. This was simply due to my extreme eyestrain. In spite of this my vision steadily improved by palming, so that at the end of three weeks I could read the 10/15 line instead of the 20/70 line. I had only an occasional eye ache when I had forgotten to use my eyes properly.

In improving my near vision, I had to make several visits to Dr. Bates, and he overcame most of my difficulties at once. I used many of the methods he advocates in this near work, but it was about three months before I could read fine print. It seemed an extremely long, long time to give up reading, but knowing now the advantages after an experience of two years without glasses, I would be willing to go without reading for a much longer period. Many people of the same age get results in a much shorter time than I did. I feel more and more strongly that a person will not have full control of his mental faculties until he gets rid of his glasses. Whether it takes two weeks or two years, the result will pay for the deprivation.

At present I usually read an hour or so in the daytime and three or four hours at night with no eyestrain whatever. Previously I used to walk along with my eyes fixed on the pavement because of the discomfort in taking note of passing people or objects; now it is a great pleasure to examine things minutely. In my work I can go nine hours with about the same fatigue as I felt before in three or four hours. In other words, Dr. Bates' work has changed me from an old man of forty-eight to a young man of fifty. I now enjoy the practice of medicine for the first time since finishing my hospital internship, as I am absolutely certain that if patients will carry out my directions their whole condition will be improved.[69]

# Old Age Sight

by William H. Bates, M.D.

[8]
When most people with normal eyes arrive at the age of forty and upwards, they usually have difficulty in reading books or newspapers, although their sight for distance may be normal. At the age of fifty or upwards, such persons become less able to read at the near point or find it impossible to read even headlines of a newspaper clearly or distinctly. This condition has been called old age sight, although it could be defined more accurately as the imperfect sight of middle age. The medical term for this form of imperfect sight is Presbyopia. While imperfect sight occurs quite commonly in middle age, it does occur in individuals under thirty years of age and more rarely in children. There are people, however, who even at the age of eighty or ninety are able to read just as well as when they were younger.

The cause of presbyopia is said to be due to the hardening of the crystalline lens of the eye to such an extent that the focus of the eye cannot be brought to a near point on account of the inability of the hard lens to change its shape. Almost every eye specialist believes this theory. In my book "Perfect Sight Without Glasses" I have described the evidence which proves that this theory is wrong.

At one time I was unable to read without glasses. After I found that the lens was not a factor in accommodation, I realized that presbyopia might be cured in some cases. Then, having cured my own eyes, I felt that the old theory of the cause of presbyopia was wrong. Since that time so many patients who were unable to read without glasses have recovered that I feel most, if not all, can be cured. In my experience I have never met with a case of presbyopia which could not be temporarily benefited.

...

Some years ago a woman, eighty-seven years old, was treated for presbyopia. The eyestrain was so great that she had been unable to obtain glasses which were satisfactory. There was a history of attacks of hemorrhage in various parts of the retina, including the region of the centre of sight or the macula. At this time, however, the hemorrhages had all disappeared, and the retina was normal.

She was very much worried about her eyes and had a lot to say. Never in my life have I heard anyone talk so rapidly and say so much in so short a time. She repeated herself over and over again, and the constant idea that she tried to emphasize was that she was blind and that no one could give her any relief. It was difficult for me to persuade her to listen to me at first. I had to wait until she stopped for breath and then I handed her some diamond type, which I asked her to read. She very promptly told me that it was impossible, that the print was too small, and that when she tried to read it she suffered from pain, headache, and discomfort.

When my second chance came to speak, I asked her to imagine the white spaces between the lines to be perfectly white. She at once told me that that would not help her, that she could put all the white between the lines that I desired and that she was confident it would not be of any use, although she claimed to have a wonderful imagination. It seemed as though I heard two voices at the same time. One was constantly repeating that it was impossible to read such fine print, while the other voice was reading it at the same time. The audience which had collected around her, relatives, friends and servants, were thrilled, and it seemed everybody was trying to say something, to offer suggestions, and to give advice. Before we could stop her, this elderly woman read the whole card as rapidly as any one could have read it who had normal vision. When she had finished reading, and while she was wondering how she came to do it, I asked her for an explanation. She answered:

"When you asked me to imagine the white spaces between the lines to be perfectly white, I at once recalled white paint. With the help of my imagination I painted these white spaces with this white paint, and when I did that I was able to read."[71]

# Stories from the Clinic ~ Presbyopia

by Emily C. Lierman

[7]

I have recently had a few cases of presbyopia which were cured in a short time. One was a woman sixty-three years of age who did fine sewing for her livelihood. She had worn glasses for more than thirty years and during the past two years her eye specialist found it difficult to fit her with glasses correctly. She had purchased her last pair the day before she came to me, and told me they made her so nervous and irritable that she could not possibly wear them more than half a day.

Her vision for the distance was normal, 15/15 with each eye separately. I gave her a small test card to hold, which has the fundamentals by Dr. W. H. Bates on the opposite side and asked her to read what she could on it. She held it at arm's length and said that she knew there was some kind of print on the card but could not tell what it was. In despair she looked at me and said, "I fear you will have a hard time getting me to read this." I gave her the small booklet containing the microscopic type and also a small card with diamond type. I placed the booklet at the lower part of the fundamental card and the diamond type card in the center. She was told to hold these about twelve inches from her eyes and not to worry about reading the print. The patient looked at me in a blank sort of way wondering how it was possible to cure presbyopia in this manner.

As she was optimistic it was easy for me to treat her. She was willing to believe that I could do for her what had been done for others whom she knew had been cured by Dr. Bates. I told her to look at the small white spaces between the lines of print in the booklet, close both eyes and remember the white spaces. She could remember them white with her eyes closed. I then told her to open her eyes and again look at the white spaces. She said they appeared whiter than they had the first time. Again I told her to close her eyes and remember the white spaces and to open them in less than a second, look at the white spaces of the diamond type card, close her eyes and remember the white spaces; then for just a second to open her eyes and look at the white spaces of the fundamental card. I told her to keep this up while I was out of the room and left her to herself for almost a half hour. Before leaving I warned her about trying to read the print, telling her that she was to flash only the white spaces.

When I returned she looked at me very much frightened and said "What am I to do, I cannot help but tell you the truth, I can read this fundamental card. I noticed that she held the fundamental card eight inches from her eyes instead of twelve. She read one sentence after another for me. I told her to be careful about staring at the type and be sure to look at the white space directly below the sentence she was reading instead of at the letters. After reading a sentence of the fundamental card she would shift to the white spaces of the blue booklet and then to the spaces of the small card and back again to the fundamental card. The treatment lasted about one hour. I told her to telephone me the next day and let me know if she had forgotten what I had directed her to do. She called and said that she was able to read some of the Bible type as well as all of the print on the fundamental card. Having read my book before she came for treatment, she knew that staring produced much discomfort and realized that she should blink frequently. Her knowledge of the benefits of blinking helped her to be cured more quickly than the usual case of this kind. The last time that she telephoned she reported that her sewing was much easier to do. She has entirely discarded her glasses and promises never to wear them again.

The second patient was a man fifty-eight years of age, a bank teller. He had heard of a bank president who had been cured by Dr. Bates. Then he obtained my book and Dr. Bates' book, "Perfect Sight Without Glasses," from the public library. He understood the directions described in each book, but there were times when he was unsuccessful in getting good results, so he came to me for help.

His sight was tested for the distance and he read 15/30 with each eye separately, although he saw some of the letters double. He complained of headache and pain in the back of his eyes, especially while working. He was then directed to palm and to imagine that he was adding accounts. He said it caused more strain and discomfort in his head and eyes. He said that it would be impossible to palm during business hours. I told him that it would not be necessary, that there were other things that he could do to prevent his headaches and eyestrain. I taught him to blink and shift all day long like the normal eye does in order to keep the eyes relaxed and in good condition. He was told to remember something perfectly, easily and without effort. He said he could remember the ocean with the tide coming in and that every seventh wave was the largest. Knowing the game of football helped him to imagine the size, color and shape of the ball. All these little details which improved his memory helped to relax his mind while his eyes were closed.

After ten minutes, he was instructed to stand with his feet about one foot apart and sway his body to the right and then to the left. As the window was close by, I directed him to look off in the distance and notice objects moving with his body, eyes and head, while things up close seemed to move opposite. He said he was hoping I would let him do that for quite a while because the bad headache he had just before coming to me, was disappearing. Then I told him to keep up the swing, looking out of the window and then toward the test card. As soon as he saw a letter I told him to look away, keeping up the swing all the while. This time he read 15/10 with each eye separately. When I gave him the fundamental card to read, he could see only sentence No. 2. All the rest of the card was very much blurred to him. Again I directed him to stand and swing and notice distant objects moving with his eyes and body, while things close appeared to move opposite.

I then had him sit in a chair with his back to the sun and told him to remember the sway of the body with his eyes closed. In a short time he began to practice again with the fundamental card, and this time he read up to No. 6 by imagining the white spaces whiter than they really were. I watched him as he tried to read further and when he began to read the small type, he stopped the blinking unconsciously and stared at the print. I noticed that his forehead became wrinkled and that he squeezed his eyes almost shut to read. I stopped this and asked him to close his eyes quickly and tell me how he felt. He had produced a strain that caused his head and eyes to ache. I reminded him that by squeezing his eyes and staring and making an effort, a strain had been produced. While his eyes were covered with the palm of one hand, he remarked, "Now I realize what I must do all day long to see without straining." I told him that when patients found out for themselves that staring brings on tension and pain, they are cured much more quickly than others who do not realize this fact. He was cured in three visits.

My third case of presbyopia, which took the longest time to cure, was a music teacher forty-nine years of age. It was very hard to convince her that I could benefit her. Her vision for the test card with each eye was normal, 15/15. When I gave her the fundamental card to read, she was quite positive that she would never read any of it without her glasses. I gave her a "Better Eyesight" magazine and told her to look at the title. She said that she could see it, but that the type was blurred as she held it at arm's length from her eyes.

She was told to close her eyes and palm with one hand and remember one of the letters of the test card that she had read at fifteen feet. Then, in less than a moment's time, I told her to remove her hand from her eyes and look at the white spaces of the fundamental card. She did this a few times and then began to smile. She said the print was beginning to clear up, but that it soon faded away and she became unable to read it again. When I told her to avoid looking at the type, she laughed. Immediately I became convinced that this was the way she read her sheet music. She looked directly at the notes and lowered her vision by staring. By closing her eyes and remembering white spaces, then opening them and looking at the white spaces, words began to clear up and she became a very different person. When she was successful in doing as I directed, she read up to No. 3 of the fundamental card. I saw her once a week for more than a month before she was able to read the entire fundamental card, eight inches from her eyes. She was told to place the small black test card on the piano near the sheet music and to frequently flash a letter of the card; then read her music. In this way she was cured. All patients cannot be treated in the same way, no matter what trouble they may have with their eyes. Eyestrain has a great deal to do with the mind and the Bates Method has surely proved it.[70]

## Central Fixation

[8] The cure of presbyopia is accomplished by eye training which secures central fixation. The patients are taught to regard the letters of the Snellen test card, the smaller letters first at ten or twenty feet, in such a way that they see a small part of each letter blacker or more distinct than the rest of the letter.

After normal vision is obtained for distance, the eye training is continued for small letters at the reading distance. A period or comma is selected. The patient regards a letter near the period or looks further away until he can appreciate that the period is less black or worse. He then regards a letter nearer the period. The distance from the period is shortened, until by practice the patient can make the period appear less black by regarding a point but a very short distance away, the diameter of a small letter. He can now read the print.

Then he is encouraged to practice holding the fine print closer to his eyes until he can read at four inches Jaeger No. 1.[72]

Some patients are relieved in a few days. Permanent relief is never obtained, without constant or daily practice, reading diamond type without glasses at four inches to twenty inches. Patients sixty, seventy, and eighty years of age have obtained relief in a short time. The efficiency of the eye is very much increased, and one reads more rapidly than with glasses and without pain or fatigue.[73]

William H. Bates, M.D.

## Central Fixation

[6] The cure of presbyopia is accomplished by eye training which secures central fixation. The patients are taught to regard the letters of the Snellen test card, the smaller letters first at ten or twenty feet, in such a way that they see a small part of each letter blacker or more distinct than the rest of the letter.

After normal vision is obtained for distance, the eye training is continued for small letters at the reading distance. A period or comma is selected. The patient regards a letter near the period or looks further away until he can appreciate that the period is less black or worse. He then regards a letter nearer the period. The distance from the period is shortened, until by practice the patient can make the period appear less black by regarding a point but a very short distance away, the diameter of a small letter. He can now read the print.

Then he is encouraged to practice holding the fine print closer to his eyes until he can read at four inches Jaeger No. 1.*

Some patients are relieved in a few days. Permanent relief is never obtained, without constant or daily practice, reading diamond type without glasses at four inches to twenty inches. Patients sixty, seventy, and eighty years of age have obtained relief in a short time. The efficiency of the eye is very much increased, and one reads more rapidly than with glasses and without pain or fatigue.

William H. Bates, M.D.

## Central Fixation

[4] The cure of presbyopia is accomplished by eye training which secures central fixation. The patients are taught to regard the letters of the Snellen test card, the smaller letters first at ten or twenty feet, in such a way that they see a small part of each letter blacker or more distinct than the rest of the letter.

After normal vision is obtained for distance, the eye training is continued for small letters at the reading distance. A period or comma is selected. The patient regards a letter near the period or looks further away until he can appreciate that the period is less black or worse. He then regards a letter nearer the period. The distance from the period is shortened, until by practice the patient can make the period appear less black by regarding a point but a very short distance away, the diameter of a small letter. He can now read the print.

Then he is encouraged to practice holding the fine print closer to his eyes until he can read at four inches Jaeger No. 1.*

Some patients are relieved in a few days. Permanent relief is never obtained, without constant or daily practice, reading diamond type without glasses at four inches to twenty inches. Patients sixty, seventy, and eighty years of age have obtained relief in a short time. The efficiency of the eye is very much increased, and one reads more rapidly than with glasses and without pain or fatigue.

William H. Bates, M.D.

# Resources

**Website links.** For links to the various internet pages listed in this book please visit www.visionsofjoy.org

**Books.** Various compilations of the best of Dr. Bates' writings have been published by Visions of Joy. These books are useful to anyone who is going through the process of improving vision naturally. All are available at www.visionsofjoy.org.

**Paperback and E-book:**

- **Bates Method Nuggets.**
  The Fundamentals of Natural Vision Improvement by Dr. W.H. Bates.
  22 chapters, 128 pages. Compiled by Esther Joy van der Werf.

**E-books:**

- **Better Eyesight.**
  The complete and searchable collection of Dr. Bates' monthly magazines,
  All 132 magazines, 771 pages. Compiled by Esther Joy van der Werf.

**"Bates Method View"-series.** E-books in this series are collections of Dr. Bates' writings on specific vision challenges. Each e-book also includes a summary of the methods used by Dr. Bates in overcoming that challenge. All are compiled by Esther Joy van der Werf.

- **The Bates Method View of Presbyopia**
- **The Bates Method View of Cataracts**
- **The Bates Method View of Conical Cornea**
- **The Bates Method View of Floating Specks**
- **The Bates Method View of Glaucoma**
- **The Bates Method View of Nystagmus**
- **The Bates Method View of Retinitis Pigmentosa**
- **Eye Education in our Schools**

**Other publications**:

- **Miniature Bibles** with microprint (available from www.visionsofjoy.org).
- More vision improvement books by other authors are listed on www.visionsofjoy.org.

**Other methods that may help you prevent and reverse presbyopia:**

- **Ray Gottlieb,** O.D., Ph.D., developed a method based on this Bates Method yet takes it a step further for presbyopia. His program for reversing presbyopia is called: "The Read Without Glasses Method." This can be purchased from www.withoutglasses.com.

  Dr. Ray Gottlieb has been an optometrist for nearly forty years with a specialty in behavioral optometry and vision therapy. He has worked at three optometry colleges and a medical school and has been the dean of the College of Syntonic Optometry since 1984. He eliminated his myopia using Bates' practices in 1972. His Ph.D. dissertation, *A Psychoneurology of Nearsightedness* (1978), explored Bates' approach to vision and myopia reduction.

  Dr. Gottlieb developed the exercises behind *The Read Without Glasses Method* in his private practice in 1976. His book: *Attention and Memory Training: Stress-Point Learning on the Trampoline* was published in 2005. Dr. Gottlieb writes and presents workshops and lectures on Bates, presbyopia, visual attention training and syntonics (optometric phototherapy). In the summers he applies his vision training to improve learning skills of advanced piano students at the Chautauqua Institution in New York.

- **Sarah Cobb** has been researching the effect of color light therapy (syntonics) on presbyopia and the results so far are promising.

  Sarah Cobb's thirty-five years in the vision field has included working as an optometric vision therapist, editor of two journals of the field of colored light therapy, administrator for the College of Syntonic Optometry, and eventually development of AcuLight Vision Enhancement, a system that addresses the underlying cause of vision problems using specific frequencies on light of acupoints around the eyes and on the body. First she addressed her own presbyopia condition by improving one diopter within the first three months of light therapy. At the age of sixty-four, she has no more need for reading glasses. During the past decade she has taught workshops around the world on a variety of vision topics which will now include presbyopia relief. She can be contacted at eyeamsarah@hotmail.com.

# Chapter Notes

[12]

**Introduction**

1. For a list of Natural Vision Educators go to www.visionsofjoy.org.

**Have Your Arms Become Too Short?**

2. Kasthurirangan, S., Glasser, A. Age related changes in accommodative dynamics in humans. *Vision Research* 46, 1507-1519, 2006.
3. Marg, Elwin. An Investigation of Voluntary as Distinguished from Reflex Accommodation. A paper read before the San Francisco Bay chapter, American Academy of Optometry, Berkeley, California, May 24, 1951.
4. Charman, W. Neil. The eye in focus: accommodation and presbyopia. *Clinical and Experimental Optometry*, 2008; 91: 3: 207-225.
5. Strenk, Susan A. et al. Age-Related Changes in Human Ciliary Muscle and Lens: A Magnetic Resonance Imaging Study. *Investigative Ophthalmology & Visual Science*, May 1999, Vol. 40, No. 6.
6. Miranda, M.N. The geographic factor in the onset of presbyopia. *Tr. Am. Ophth. Soc.* Vol LXXVII, 1979.
7. Eskridge, Jess B. Review of Ciliary Muscle Effort in Presbyopia. *American Journal of Optometry & Physiological Optics*, Vol 61, No.2, pp. 133-138.
8. Stieve, R. Über den Bau des menschlichen Ciliarmuskels, seine Veränderungen während des Lebens und seine Bedeutung für die Akkommodation. *Anatomischer Anzeiger* 97, 69-79 (1945). (As cited in Atchinson, 1995, see note 15.)
9. Weale, R.A. *A Biography of the Eye*, H.K. Lewis, London, UK (1982). (As cited in Atchinson, 1995, see note 15.)
10. Donders, F.C. On the anomalies of accommodation and refraction of the eye. London: New Sydenham Soc., 1864. (As cited in Pierscionek, 1993, see note 16.)
11. Duane, A. Are the current theories of accommodation correct? *Am J Ophthalmol* 1925; 8: 196-202. (As cited in Pierscionek, 1993, see note 16.)
12. Farnsworth, P.N. and Shyne, S.E. Anterior zonular shifts with age. *Exp. Eye Res.* 28, 291-297 (1979). (As cited in Atchinson, 1995, see note 15.)

13. Buschmann, W., Linnert, D., Hofman, W. and Gross, A. Die Reissfestigkeit der menschlichen Zonula and ihre Abhänggigkeit vom Lebensalter. *Graefes Arch. Klin. Exp. Ophthalmol.* 206, 183-190 (1978). (As cited in Atchinson, 1995, see note 15.)
14. Weale, Robert, D.Sc. Presbyopia Toward the End of the 20th Century. *Survey of Ophthalmology*, Volume 34, number 1, July-August 1989.
15. Atchinson, D.A. Accommodation and presbyopia. *Ophthal. Physiol. Opt.* Vol 15, No. 4, pp. 255-272, 1995.
16. Pierscionek, Barbara K., Ph.D. What we know and understand about presbyopia. *Clinical & Experimental Optometry* 76.3, 1993 May/June.
17. Burke, A.G. et al. Population-Based Study of Presbyopia in Rural Tanzania. *Ophthalmology 2006*; 113:723-727, 2006.
18. Presbyopia; Its Cause and Cure: Bates, William H., M.D., *Perfect Sight Without Glasses*, Central Fixation Publishing Company, New York City, 1920, Chapter 20, page 218.
19. Vedamurthy, I. et al. The Influence of First Near-Spectacle Reading Correction on Accommodation and Its Interaction with Convergence. *Invest. Ophthalmol. Vis. Sci.*; 50(9): 4215-4222, September 2009.
20. Reading: Bates, William H., M.D., *Better Eyesight*, Central Fixation Publishing Company, New York City, May 1926.

**Step 1. Meet Your Blurry Vision**

21. Vedamurthy, Influence of Frist Near-Spectacle Reading Correction, 2009
22. Cured of presbyopia in his early fifties: Bates, *Better Eyesight*, February 1922.
23. Old Age Sight: Bates, *Better Eyesight*, June 1925.
24. Discard Glasses: Bates, *Better Eyesight*, June 1922
25. To find a behavioral optometrist near you check www.visionsofjoy.org.
26. Affordable prescription glasses can be bought online. See www.visionsofjoy.org.
27. Pinhole glasses: See www.visionsofjoy.org.
28. Example of strain recognized early: Bates, *Better Eyesight*, April 1921.

**Step 2. Time for a Good Rest**

29. Couple cured by closing eyes: Bates, *Better Eyesight*, April 1921.
30. Cure only without effort: Bates, *Better Eyesight*, March 1926.
31. Ott, John. *Health and Light* and *Light, Radiation and You* and *My Ivory Cellar*
32. Fear of light: Bates, *Better Eyesight*, December 1921.
33. A 250W incandescent light bulb is comparable (in lumens at least) to a 55W compact fluorescent light (CFL). An incandescent light's spectrum is closer to sunlight and therefore preferable over CFLs.
    French research cautions against using LED lights due to risks for health and eyesight. You can read the article at www.visionsofjoy.org. Until further research is done it may be wise to restrict the use of LEDs as much as possible.
34. Darkness is dangerous: Bates, *Perfect Sight Without Glasses*, 1920, page 189.
35. Taken from "Chinese Acupuncture Points for the Eyes," a chart by the late Deborah Banker, M.D., which she gave out during her lecture at the North American Vision Conference of 2004.
36. Forrest, Elliott B., O.D. Astigmatism as a Function of Visual Scan, Head Scan, and Head Posture. *American Journal of Optometry & Physiological Optics*, Vol. 57, No. 11, p844-860, November 1980.
37. Weale, Robert, D.Sc. Presbyopia Toward the End of the 20th Century. *Survey of Ophthalmology*, Volume 34, number 1, July-August 1989.
38. "Worldwide Distribution of Visual Refractive Errors and What to Expect at a Particular Location" Presentation to the *International Society for Geographic and Epidemiologic Ophthalmology* by David W. Dunaway and Dr. Ian Berger. (Also presented at the Affordable Vision Correction Conference by Dr. Ian Berger and Dr. K. Mistry, 7-9 August 2004, University of Oxford, UK, http://www.affordable-vision-correction.org/prog.html).
39. Remember your successes: Bates, *Better Eyesight*, December 1921.

**Step 3. Start on Easy Street**

40. Examples of full spectrum lamps are at www.visionsofjoy.org.
41. Drink enough water: Bates, Emily, *Better Eyesight*, June 1929
42. Weale, Presbyopia toward the end of the 20th century, 1989, p19.

43. Sardi, Bill. *Nutrition and the eyes: How to keep your eyes healthy naturally.* Vol.I, Health Spectrum Publishers, 1994, p65.

44. Anshel, Jeffrey, O.D. *Smart medicine for your eyes: A guide to safe and effective relief of common eye disorders.* Avery Publishing Group, Garden City Park, NY, 1999, p188.

45. Kaplan, Robert-M., O.D. *The power behind your eyes: Improving your eyesight with integrated vision therapy*. Healing Arts Press, Rochester, Vermont, 1995, Table 2, p153.

**Step 4. Near Vision Warm-Ups**

46. Weale, Robert Alexander D.Sc. Epidemiology of refractive errors and presbyopia. *Survey of Ophthalmology*, Vol 28, Issue 5, September-October 2003, p515-543.

**Step 5. Get into the Swing**

47. SwingWindows software (for PC only) can be downloaded at www.visionsofjoy.org

**Step 7. Holy Halos!**

48. Halos (top quote): Bates, *Better Eyesight*, January 1925.

49. Halos: Bates, *Better Eyesight*, February 1920 and March 1925.

**Step 8. Guidance from a Bright White Line**

50. The thin white line: Bates, *Better Eyesight*, August 1928, May and July 1929.

51. Failure to read fine print: Bates, *Better Eyesight*, May 1926 and May 1929.

52. Thin white line: Bates, *Better Eyesight*, January 1930.

53. Speed reading: Bates, *Better Eyesight*, October 1926.

**Step 9. Love the Fine Print**

54. Fine print: Bates, *Better Eyesight*, May 1920.

55. Seven Truths of Normal Sight: Bates, *Better Eyesight*, May 1920.

**Step 10. Read Disclaimers by Candlelight**

56. Fine print under unfavorable conditions: Bates, *Better Eyesight*, June 1921.
57. A little research I did revealed that typography and its font sizes are not an exact science… Fonts have names, such as brilliant, diamond, pearl, nonpareille, garamond, pica, etc. Originally each of these names represented a specific font size, with nonpareille equal to half pica, and garamond being double pearl. In the $17^{th}$ and $18^{th}$ century efforts to standardize font sizes in typography led to a common measurement: 'printer points'. An inch has 72 points.
    In *The Practice of Typography* by Theodore Low DeVinne (1914) diamond is listed as 4.5 points, yet in the mid 1800s diamond was either 4.1, 4.2 or 4.3 points depending on which foundry you asked. (Sources: William Savage, *Dictionary of Printing*, 1842, page 802. *Printer's Miscellany*, New York, July 1857.)
    In addition to these slight differences, the actual size of a printer's point also varied as printers in France, The Netherlands, England, Germany and the United States developed their own systems.
    To add to the confusion, Dr. Bates equated diamond to jaeger 1 in "Treatment of Myopia without Glasses" (an article published in *The Medical Record*, January 27, 1894, p104-106). According to *Near Visual Acuity Tests* by M. Sachsenweger (1987, p24) jaeger 1 is equivalent to 3 printer points. (Also see note 72 below.)
    Instead of trying to determine the true size of diamond, if there is such a thing, I chose to just get close to the "Specimen of Diamond Type" printed on page 195 of Dr. Bates' 1920 book *Perfect Sight Without Glasses*. The 5 point times new roman font I use for diamond is close to the 4 point size in Sachsenweger's book, it may even be 4.5 points, but that is 'beside the point' as it serves its intended purpose. I trust you will agree.
58. Relaxation from fine print: Bates, *Better Eyesight*, May 1922.
59. Memory and imagination to read diamond print: Bates, *Better Eyesight*, September 1924.
60. *The Practice of Typography* by Theodore Low DeVinne mentions on page 68 that Henri Didot, a printer in Paris, created a 2.5 point font in 1827 that he called "microscopique." The font used in this book for microscopic print is times new roman 2 point, which is slightly larger than the microscopic print shown on page 195 of *Perfect Sight Without Glasses*.
61. Using microscopic print: Bates, *Better Eyesight*, May 1926.

**Throw Away Your Reading Glasses**

62. Things we stop doing: Bates, *Better Eyesight*, April 1927.

**Inspirational Stories**

63. From the author's personal correspondence with Trudy Eyges, May-July 2013.
64. Prevention of Presbyopia is Easy: Bates, *Better Eyesight*, April 1927.
65. Presbyopia; Its Cause and Cure: Bates, *Perfect Sight Without Glasses*, Chapter 20.
66. Effects of Presbyopia: Bates, *Better Eyesight*, May 1926.
67. Fine Print: Bates, *Better Eyesight*, April 1927.
68. Stories from the Clinic – Three Cases of Presbyopia: Bates, *Better Eyesight*, April 1921.
69. An Oculist's Experience: Darling, E.F., M.D., *Better Eyesight*, December 1925
70. Old Age Sight: Bates, *Better Eyesight*, June 1925.
71. Stories from the Clinic – Presbyopia: Bates, *Better Eyesight*, April 1927.
72. Jaeger 1 has a typographic measurement of N-3, which is this size:

    This is jaeger 1. ~ Your goal is to read this without glasses. Yes, you can! Relaxed practice makes perfect…

    When you can read jaeger 1 at twelve inches (thirty cm) from your eyes your near vision acuity is 100%, or the equivalent of 20/20 distance vision. The third text box on page 116 is printed in times new roman 4 point font, equivalent to jaeger 1.
73. Central Fixation: Bates, William H., M.D., *New York Medical Journal,* May 8, 1915.

**Glossary**

74. Central Fixation definition: Bates, William H., M.D., *New York Medical Journal,* February 3, 1917.

# Practice Charts

In medical dictionaries an eye chart is defined as "a chart read at a fixed distance for purposes of testing sight." Think about that for a moment. When your sight is "tested" under rigid conditions, chances are that you will try hard and strain to 'pass' this test. You now know that straining to see is unlikely to give you the results you want.

What if you start from a different perspective? Instead of using the term "eye chart", I prefer to use the term "practice chart." You practice staying relaxed with these charts; you do not test your sight with them. The better you become at viewing these charts in a relaxed way, the more the letters will appear as they truly are – distinct, black and easy to read.

This section has several practice charts and near vision cards. These are intended to be cut out along the dotted lines and used alongside the book.

[15] **How to use a practice chart to monitor your progress**
Depending on your initial level of vision, use either the small or medium practice chart at a distance of one foot (twelve inches or thirty cm) from the eyes. If the entire chart is very blurry at that point, hold the chart at the distance where you can read most of the chart easily (four or five lines) without your glasses. Measure that distance from your eyes.

After you checked your acuity with both eyes open, cover the right eye with your right hand and note the acuity for the left eye. Go back to using both eyes for a few moments before you cover the left eye with your left hand to check the acuity for the right eye. (It does not matter in which order you check your eyes.) Write your results in the table on page 128.

You can record your visual acuity as follows: write the distance (in feet) where you held the practice chart before the slash ( / ). After the slash write the number that you find next to the last line of letters that you were able to read. Here is an example:

Jane holds the chart one foot from her eyes. With both eyes open she is able to read most of the line that has the number 5 next to it. She writes down her vision acuity for both eyes as **1 / 5**. At that same distance, with her right eye covered, her left eye can only read the letters on the 7 line, but not those on the 5 line, so her left eye's acuity is written as **1 / 7**. When she switches over and covers her left eye, (giving her right eye a few moments to re-adjust) she reads the 5 line, but not yet the 4 line, so her right eye on its own has **1 / 5** acuity.

If Jane recognizes one letter on the 4 line but not the rest, she can specify that by writing **1 / 5** $^{+1}$. If she misses one letter on the 5 line and correctly recognizes the others on that line she writes **1 / 5** $^{-1}$.

The font sizes of the lines on the practice charts are provided below.

Someone with normal near vision is able to read the 1 line from one foot, but many people can do even better and read that 1 line from six inches or even from four inches.

**Practice chart letter sizes**

| Line on chart: | Arial Bold Font size: |
|---|---|
| 200 | 355 |
| 100 | 177 |
| 80 | 142 |
| 50 | 89 |
| 40 | 71 |
| 30 | 53 |
| 25 | 44.5 |
| 20 | 35.5 |
| 15 | 26.5 |
| 10 | 17.5 |
| 7 | 12.5 |
| 5 | 9 |
| 4 | 7 |
| 3 | 5.5 |
| 2 | 4.5 |
| 1 | 3 |

## Your Visual Acuity Record Sheet

**Record your progress**

Once per week record your vision acuity below. Your vision can be quite different at night under artificial light than in the daytime in bright sunlight, so always make a note of the light conditions. If you know what the light conditions were, you can make a fair comparison week to week. For example, if one week you check your vision at noon while the sun shines brightly, but the next week, also at noon, it is heavily overcast outside, you will understand if the result of the second week is not as good as the first week.

**Visual Acuity**

| Date | Time | Both Eyes | Left Eye | Right Eye | Light conditions |
|---|---|---|---|---|---|
| | | / | / | / | |
| | | / | / | / | |
| | | / | / | / | |
| | | / | / | / | |
| | | / | / | / | |
| | | / | / | / | |
| | | / | / | / | |
| | | / | / | / | |
| | | / | / | / | |
| | | / | / | / | |
| | | / | / | / | |
| | | / | / | / | |
| | | / | / | / | |
| | | / | / | / | |
| | | / | / | / | |
| | | / | / | / | |

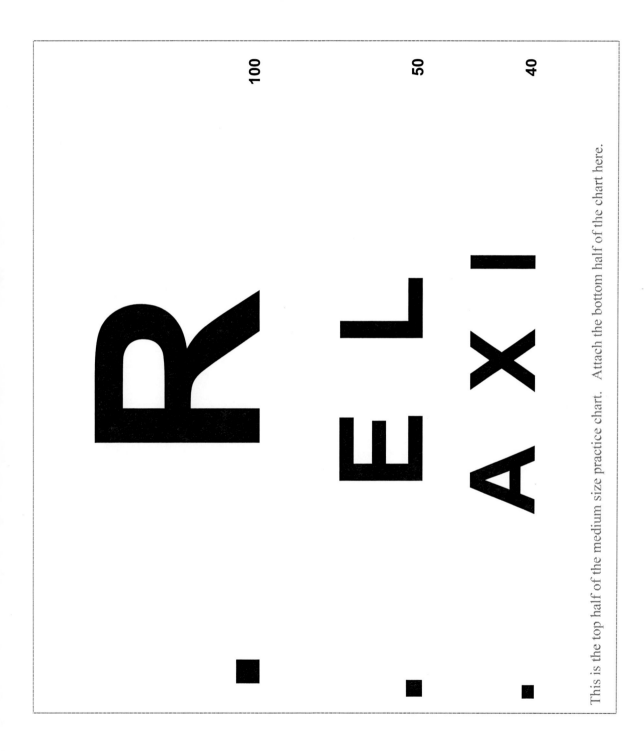


This is the top half of the medium size practice chart. Attach the bottom half of the chart here.

Read Without Glasses at Any Age
by Esther Joy van der Werf
www.visionsofjoy.org

This is the bottom half of the medium size practice chart. Attach the top half of the chart here.

| | | |
|---|---|---|
| . | N T O S | 25 |
| . | E E I N G | 20 |
| . | C E N T R A L | 15 |
| . | C L A R I T Y | 10 |
| . | S H I F T B L I | 7 |
| . | N K A N D B R E A T H E | 5 |
| . | © 2013 VISIONS OF JOY • NATURAL VISION PRACTICE CHART. | 3 |

Read Without Glasses at Any Age
by Esther Joy van der Werf
www.visionsofjoy.org

## Two Near Vision Practice Charts

R 20
E L 15
A X I 10
N T O S 7
E E I N G 5
C E N T R A L 4
C L A R I T Y 3
S H I F T B L I 2
N K A N D B R E A T H E 1

© 2013 VISIONS OF JOY • NATURAL VISION PRACTICE CHART FOR NEAR VISION.

R 20
E L 15
A X I 10
N T O S 7
E E I N G 5
C E N T R A L 4
C L A R I T Y 3
S H I F T B L I 2
N K A N D B R E A T H E 1

© 2013 VISIONS OF JOY • NATURAL VISION PRACTICE CHART FOR NEAR VISION.

Read Without Glasses at Any Age
by Esther Joy van der Werf
www.visionsofjoy.org

Read Without Glasses at Any Age
by Esther Joy van der Werf
www.visionsofjoy.org

# Fundamentals

by W.H. Bates, M.D.

1. Glasses discarded permanently.

2. Central Fixation is seeing best where you are looking.

3. Favorable conditions: Light may be bright or dim. The distance of the print from the eyes, where seen best, also varies with people.

4. Shifting: With normal sight the eyes are moving all the time.

5. Swinging: When the eyes move slowly or rapidly from side to side, stationary objects appear to move in the opposite direction.

6. Long Swing: Stand with the feet about one foot apart, turn the body to the right – at the same time lifting the heel of the left foot. Do not move the head or eyes or pay any attention to the apparent movement of stationary objects. Now place the left heel on the floor, turn the body to the left, raising the heel of the right foot. Alternate.

7. Drifting Swing: When practicing this swing, one pays no attention to the clearness of stationary objects, which appear to be moving. The eyes wander from point to point slowly, easily, or lazily, so that the stare or strain may be avoided.

8. Variable Swing: Hold the forefinger of one hand six inches from the right eye and about the same distance to the right, look straight ahead and move the head a short distance from side to side. The finger appears to move.

9. Stationary Objects Moving: By moving the head and eyes a short distance from side to side, being sure to blink, one can imagine stationary objects to be moving.

10. Memory: Improving the memory of letters and other objects improves the vision for everything.

11. Imagination: We see only what we think we see, or what we imagine. We can only imagine what we remember.

12. Rest: All cases of imperfect sight are improved by closing the eyes and resting them.

13. Palming: The closed eyes may be covered with the palm of one or both hands.

14. Blinking: The normal eye blinks, or closes and opens very frequently.

15. Mental Pictures: As long as one is awake one has all kinds of memories of mental pictures. If these pictures are remembered easily, perfectly, the vision is benefited.

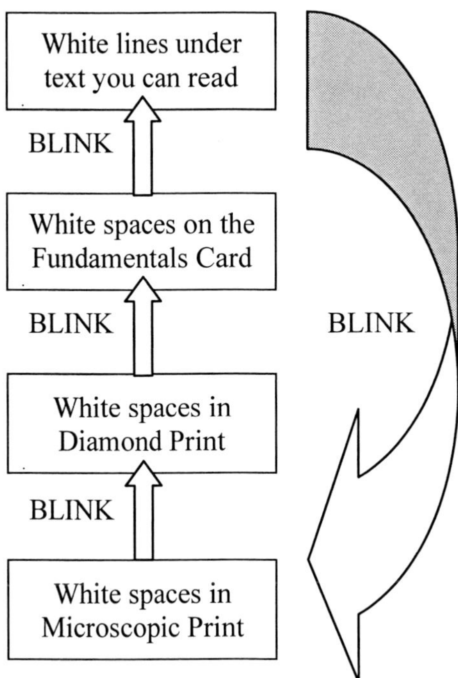


Repeat this until you can read all the lines of the Fundamental card and the diamond print.

Read Without Glasses at Any Age
by Esther Joy van der Werf
www.visionsofjoy.org

# Diamond & Microscopic Print Practice Card

Hold this card underneath the Fundamentals card on page 135
(For instructions see Step 10, pages 94-95)

Seven Truths of Normal Sight

1—Normal Sight can always be demonstrated in the normal eye, but only under favorable conditions.

2—Central Fixation: The letter or part of the letter regarded is always seen best.

3—Shifting: The point regarded changes rapidly and continuously.

4—Swinging: When the shifting is slow, the letters appear to move from side to side or in other directions with a pendulum-like motion.

5—Memory is perfect The color and background of the letters, or other objects seen are remembered perfectly, instantaneously and continuously.

6—Imagination is good. One may even see the white part of the letters whiter than it really is, while the black is not altered by distance, illumination, size, or form, of the letters.

7—Rest or relaxation of the eye and mind is perfect and can always be demonstrated.

When one of these seven fundamentals is perfect all are perfect.

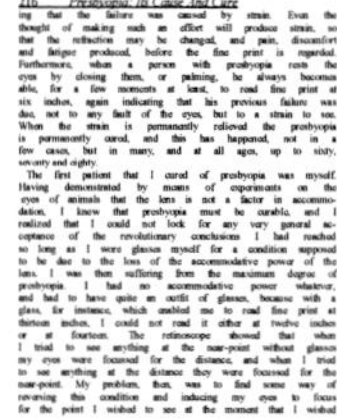

216 *Presbyopia: Its Cause And Cure*

ing that the failure was caused by strain. Even the thought of making such an effort will produce strain, so that the refraction may be changed, and pain, discomfort and fatigue produced, before the fine print is regarded. Furthermore, when a person with presbyopia rests the eyes by closing them, or palming, he always becomes able, for a few moments at least, to read fine print at six inches, again indicating that his previous failure was due, not to any fault of the eyes, but to a strain to see. When the strain is permanently relieved the presbyopia is permanently cured, and this has happened, not in a few cases, but in many, and at all ages, up to sixty, seventy and eighty.

The first patient that I cured of presbyopia was myself. Having demonstrated by means of experiments on the eyes of animals that the lens is not a factor in accommodation, I knew that presbyopia must be curable, and I realized that I could not look for any very general acceptance of the revolutionary conclusions I had reached so long as I wore glasses myself for a condition supposed to be due to the loss of the accommodative power of the lens. I was then suffering from the maximum degree of presbyopia. I had no accommodative power whatever, and had to have quite an outfit of glasses, because with a glass, for instance, which enabled me to read fine print at thirteen inches, I could not read it either at twelve inches or at fourteen. The retinoscope showed that when I tried to see anything at the near-point without glasses my eyes were focussed for the distance, and when I tried to see anything at the distance they were focussed for the near-point. My problem, then, was to find some way of reversing this condition and inducing my eyes to focus for the point I wished to see at the moment that I wished

*Only One Man Who Could Cure Me* 217

to see it. I consulted various eye specialists, but my language was to them like that of St. Paul to the Greeks, namely, foolishness. "Your lens is as hard as a stone," they said. "No one can do anything for you." Then I went to a nerve specialist. He used the retinoscope on me, and confirmed my own observations as to the peculiar contrariness of my accommodation; but he had no idea what I could do about it. He would consult some of his colleagues, he said, and asked me to come back in a month, which I did. Then he told me he had come to the conclusion that there was only one man who could cure me, and that was Dr. William H. Bates of New York.

"Why do you say that?" I asked.

"Because you are the only man who seems to know anything about it," he answered.

Thus thrown upon my own resources, I was fortunate enough to find a nonmedical gentleman who was willing to do what he could to assist me, the Rev. R. B. B. Foote, of Brooklyn. He kindly used the retinoscope through many long and tedious hours while I studied my own case, and tried to find some way of accommodating when I wanted to read, instead of when I wanted to see something at the distance. One day, while looking at a picture of the Rock of Gibraltar which hung on the wall, I noted some black spots on its face. I imagined that these spots were the openings of caves, and that there were people in these caves moving about. When I did this my eyes were focussed for the reading distance. Then I looked at the same picture at the reading distance, still imagining that the spots were caves with people in them. The retinoscope showed that I had accommodated, and I was able to read the lettering beside the picture. I had,

**Cut out this practice card and keep it in your wallet**

**Seven Truths of Normal Sight**

1—Normal Sight can always be demonstrated in the normal eye, but only under favorable conditions.

2—Central Fixation: The letter or part of the letter regarded is always seen best.

3—Shifting: The point regarded changes rapidly and continuously.

4—Swinging: When the shifting is slow, the letters appear to move from side to side or in other directions with a pendulum-like motion.

5—Memory is perfect The color and background of the letters, or other objects seen are remembered perfectly, instantaneously and continuously.

6—Imagination is good. One may even see the white part of the letters whiter than it really is, while the black is not altered by distance, illumination, size, or form, of the letters.

7—Rest or relaxation of the eye and mind is perfect and can always be demonstrated.

When one of these seven fundamentals is perfect all are perfect.

Read Without Glasses at Any Age. www.visionsofjoy.org Natural Eyesight Improvement

Read Without Glasses at Any Age
by Esther Joy van der Werf
www.visionsofjoy.org

**Microprint Practice Card**

216 *Presbyopia: Its Cause And Cure*

ing that the failure was caused by strain. Even the thought of making such an effort will produce strain, so that the refraction may be changed, and pain, discomfort and fatigue produced, before the fine print is regarded. Furthermore, when a person with presbyopia rests the eyes by closing them, or palming, he always becomes able, for a few moments at least, to read fine print at six inches, again indicating that his previous failure was due, not to any fault of the eyes, but to a strain to see. When the strain is permanently relieved the presbyopia is permanently cured, and this has happened, not in a few cases, but in many, and at all ages, up to sixty, seventy and eighty.

The first patient that I cured of presbyopia was myself. Having demonstrated by means of experiments on the eyes of animals that the lens is not a factor in accommodation, I knew that presbyopia must be curable, and I realized that I could not look for any very general acceptance of the revolutionary conclusions I had reached so long as I wore glasses myself for a condition supposed to be due to the loss of the accommodative power of the lens. I was then suffering from the maximum degree of presbyopia. I had no accommodative power whatever, and had to have quite an outfit of glasses, because with a glass, for instance, which enabled me to read fine print at thirteen inches, I could not read it either at twelve inches or at fourteen. The retinoscope showed that when I tried to see anything at the near-point without glasses my eyes were focussed for the distance, and when I tried to see anything at the distance they were focussed for the near-point. My problem, then, was to find some way of reversing this condition and inducing my eyes to focus for the point I wished to see at the moment that I wished

*Only One Man Who Could Cure Me* 217

to see it. I consulted various eye specialists, but my language was to them like that of St. Paul to the Greeks, namely, foolishness. "Your lens is as hard as a stone," they said. "No one can do anything for you." Then I went to a nerve specialist. He used the retinoscope on me, and confirmed my own observations as to the peculiar contrariness of my accommodation; but he had no idea what I could do about it. He would consult some of his colleagues, he said, and asked me to come back in a month, which I did. Then he told me he had come to the conclusion that there was only one man who could cure me, and that was Dr. William H. Bates of New York.

"Why do you say that?" I asked.

"Because you are the only man who seems to know anything about it," he answered.

Thus thrown upon my own resources, I was fortunate enough to find a nonmedical gentleman who was willing to do what he could to assist me, the Rev. R. B. B. Foote, of Brooklyn. He kindly used the retinoscope through many long and tedious hours while I studied my own case, and tried to find some way of accommodating when I wanted to read, instead of when I wanted to see something at the distance. One day, while looking at a picture of the Rock of Gibraltar which hung on the wall, I noted some black spots on its face. I imagined that these spots were the openings of caves, and that there were people in these caves moving about. When I did this my eyes were focussed for the reading distance. Then I looked at the same picture at the reading distance, still imagining that the spots were caves with people in them. The retinoscope showed that I had accommodated, and I was able to read the lettering beside the picture. I had,

Read Without Glasses at Any Age www.visionsofjoy.org Natural Eyesight Improvement

# Diamond Print Practice Cards

Read Without Glasses at Any Age ~ Diamond Print Practice Card

Step 1. **Become aware of eyestrain** and other factors that contribute to blurry vision, so you can begin to turn the tide. Stop using reading glasses or temporarily use lower-strength glasses or pinhole glasses. Accept your blurry vision; never strain to see.

Step 2. **Rest your eyes** with palming, sunning and massage. Close your eyes whenever they feel tired and keep them closed until they feel rested. Blink regularly and easily. Good posture helps to release eye muscle tension. Imagine clarity at the near point. Let images of achieving your goal of excellent vision inspire you!

Step 3. Once your eyes are rested, begin with **your most favorable conditions** in terms of light, print size, and distance. Choose inspiring texts and aim for optimal nutrition.

Step 4. **Practice seeing effortlessly at the near point** with some near-vision warm-ups using the palm of your hand or fun, colorful objects. Enjoy close encounters. Make good use of your memory and imagination.

Step 5. **Move** your head or the page and relax your neck and eye muscles through motion. Swing side to side, as well as back and forth in and out of your blur zone to invite the eyes to focus. Notice apparent motion all day long.

Step 6. **Improve your central clarity.** Practice seeing one letter best at a time, then part of a letter better than the rest of the same letter. Progress gradually from large to small print and from far to near. Avoid the tunnel vision trap with a relaxed awareness of your entire field of vision.

Step 7. When you let your eyes be the light-finders they are, you can imagine the white in and around letters to be brighter white and you will **notice halos** that make the black letters stand out darker. Here too, gradually progress from large letters to small, and use your memory and imagination.

Step 8. **Follow the thin bright white line** underneath lines of text. Let it effortlessly guide your attention along the bottom of the print. When you keep your attention mostly with the thin bright white line, reading becomes effortless. Practice with text at your optimal distances for fastest improvement.

Step 9. **Love the fine print!** Small print stimulates natural correct use of the eyes, as long as you do not strain to read it. Begin at your optimal distance and read at your normal speed as much as possible. Gradually decrease the distance at which you hold it.

Step 10. **Read disclaimers by candlelight** or at least practice relaxing with diamond print at four inches from your eyes. Make smart use of microscopic print and dim light. Let your imagination clear the print, even if it seems impossible to read. Oh, and throw away those glasses…

www.VisionsOfJoy.org

Read Without Glasses at Any Age ~ Diamond Print Practice Card

**HALOS**
by William H. Bates, M.D.

"The eyes, when reading perfectly,
do not look directly at the letters,
but at the white spaces or the halos."

When people with normal sight look at the large letters on the Snellen test card, at any distance, from twenty feet to six inches or less, they see, at the inner and outer edges and in the openings of the round letters, a white more intense than the margin of the card. Similarly, when they read fine print, the spaces between the lines and the letters and the openings of the letters appear whiter than the margin of the page, while streaks of an even more intense white may be seen along the edges of the lines of letters.

It can be demonstrated that this is an illusion. We do not see illusions; we only imagine them. When the white spaces between the lines appear whiter than the margin of the page, we call these white spaces "halos."

These "halos" are sometimes seen so vividly that in order to convince people that they are illusions it is often necessary to cover the letters, when they at once disappear.

Most of us believe we see them, and it is very difficult for many people to realize that the halos are not seen, but only imagined. The halos might be called the connecting link between imagination and sight. To see the halos is to improve the imagination, and the vision for the letters is also improved.

People with imperfect sight may also see the halos, though less perfectly, and when they understand that they are imagined, they often become able to imagine them where they had not been seen before, or to increase their vividness, in which case the sight always improves.

This can be done by imagining the appearances first with the eyes closed; and then looking at the card, or at fine print, and imagining them there. By alternating these two acts of imagination the sight is often improved rapidly.

One can improve the vision for reading not by looking at the letters, but by improving the imagination of the halos. To look at the letters very soon brings on a strain, with imperfect sight. To look at the white spaces and to improve their whiteness, is a benefit to the imagination and to the vision. One cannot read fine print at all unless the halos are imagined.

It is best to begin the practice at the point at which the halos are seen, or can be imagined best. Nearsighted people are usually able to see them at the near-point, sometimes very vividly. Farsighted people may also see them best at this point, although their sight for form may be best at the distance.

By practice one becomes able to imagine or to see the halos more perfectly — the better the imagination, the better the sight.

www.VisionsOfJoy.org

Read Without Glasses at Any Age
by Esther Joy van der Werf
www.visionsofjoy.org

Read Without Glasses at Any Age
by Esther Joy van der Werf
www.visionsofjoy.org

# Better Eyesight ~ Naturally

by Esther Joy van der Werf ~ www.visionsofjoy.org

1. Use lower diopter glasses, and only when absolutely necessary.

2. **Blink** frequently and effortlessly. Blinking cleanses, lubricates and rests the eyes while giving them the opportunity to refocus.

3. **Central fixation** is seeing best where you are looking, and allowing the eyes to continually **shift** to the next point of attention. Remain aware of peripheral vision, which is not seen as clearly as the small 'crystal ball' of central vision.

4. Close your eyes whenever they are tired. When **palming** the eyes, feel any muscle strain disappear easily from your eyelids, eyes, face and neck; then imagine already seeing clearly at any distance, effortlessly.

5. **Sunshine** on closed eyelids will help build light tolerance and reduces dependency on sunglasses. Regular sunning is excellent for vision and health. Enjoy time outside each day.

6. Allow your head to **move** along with your eyes. A tall and balanced **posture** will aid this movement and will help release neck tension.

7. **Think positive**. Look for solutions and focus on the bright side of life. A happy mind creates happy eyes.

8. Practice **reading** small print, using all the good vision habits. Follow the thin bright white line right underneath the letters. This reduces strain and relaxes the eyes. Vary the reading distance and look up regularly to briefly focus afar.

9. Improve natural abdominal **breathing** by learning to gently extend the exhale. **Relaxation** is the key to both breathing and vision.

10. Forget about your eyes; **receive** images easily by letting your brain do the seeing. You can now let go of old habits of staring, squinting or trying to see.

11. See **apparent motion**. Due to the natural shifting motion of the eyes, stationary objects appear to be moving. Imagine that you see this gentle swinging motion all day long.

12. Improving the **memory** of letters or other objects improves the vision for everything. Let your **imagination** provide even more details and clarity.

13. Gently **massage** around the eyes to stimulate acupressure points. This also improves circulation.

14. The best foods for your eyes are green leafy vegetables. Enjoy a salad or green smoothie daily

T

H I

N K P

O S I T

I V E F O

C U S O N T

H E B R I G H

T S I D E O F L I F E

L O O K F O R S O L U T I O N S

B L I N K R E G U L A R L Y A N D B R E A T H E E A S I L Y

M O V E E Y E S S W I F T L Y ☺ E N J O Y D A I L Y S U N S H I N E

P A L M W H E N T I R E D ~ R E M E M B E R T A L L P O S T U R E

ENJOY A RELAXED AWARENESS OF PERIPHERY WHILE CENTRALIZING ATTENTION

# Glossary

**Accommodation:** The automatic adjustment of the eye for seeing at different distances thought to be effected chiefly by changes in the convexity of the crystalline lens.

**Astigmatism:** An irregularly shaped eye, lens or cornea, causing rays from a point to fail to meet in a focal point on the retina resulting in a blurred and imperfect image.

**Central Fixation:** "By 'central fixation' is meant a passive, receptive, or relaxed condition of the eyes and brain. When the mind is sufficiently at rest the eye sees best the point fixed – in other words, the eye sees best what it is looking at."[74]

**Cornea:** The transparent outer layer of the eyeball at the front; the area that covers the iris and pupil.

**Ciliary Muscle:** A circular muscle situated in the ciliary body and connected to the lens by zonules. When this muscle contracts it relaxes the zonules so that the lens is permitted to become more rounded for near vision.

**Diopter:** A unit of measurement of the refractive power of a lens; it relates to the capacity of the lens to bend rays of light.

**Extraocular muscle:** Any of the six muscles attached to the outside of the eye which control the movement of the eye within the eye-socket.

**Hyperopia / Hypermetropia / Farsightedness / Long Sight:** A condition in which visual images come to a focus behind the retina of the eye and vision is better for distant than for near objects.

**Minus Lens / Concave lens:** A lens that is ground thinner in the center to improve focus for people with myopia.

**Myopia / Nearsightedness / Short Sight:** A condition in which the visual images come to a focus in front of the retina of the eye and vision is better for near than for distant objects.

**Prescription:** A written formula for the grinding of compensating lenses for glasses and contacts.

**Presbyopia / Middle Age Farsightedness:** A visual condition which becomes apparent especially in middle age and which manifests in defective accommodation and inability to focus sharply for near vision.

**Plus Lens / Convex Lens:** A lens that is ground thinner at the edges to improve focus for people with hyperopia or presbyopia.

**Retina:** The sensory membrane that lines the back of the eye. It is composed of several layers including one containing the rods and cones (our light receptor cells) which are triggered by light coming through the lens and convert that stimulus into chemical and nervous signals which reach the brain by way of the optic nerve.

**Vitreous Body:** The transparent jelly-like fluid that fills the eyeball behind the lens.

**Zonules (of Zinn):** The suspensory ligaments of the crystalline lens that hold the lens in place within the ciliary body. These ligaments also keep the lens from wobbling while you walk, and they are involved in accommodation.

# Index

## *A*



## *B*



## *C*



## *D*



## *E*



## *F*

## G



## H



## I



## L



## M



## N



## O

# About the Author

Growing up in the Netherlands Esther van der Werf enjoyed excellent eyesight until her late teens, when her vision changed to slightly myopic. A visit to an optometrist resulted in a prescription for glasses. She did not particularly like the glasses; they made her feel separate from the world – an observer rather than a participant. The glasses were more of an obstacle than a help, so she cunningly 'lost' them, to the dismay of her parents.

Over the next sixteen years Esther got used to her somewhat blurry vision. She once tried eye exercises from a book but did not notice any improvement, until, in her early thirties, she read *Relearning to See* which taught her that vision improves with relaxation, not eye exercises. This worked very well for her; within two weeks her acuity improved from 20/50 to 20/20 while color perception was also enhanced. She proceeded to test this method on a nearsighted friend whose sight also improved a lot. Thus convinced that the Bates Method was worth studying, she enrolled in Tom Quackenbush's teacher training program in San Francisco in 2000 and felt she had finally found her mission: helping others to regain their clarity as she had done.
To continue her own training she read all of Dr. Bates' materials, worked with Marc Grossman O.D., L.Ac., in New York, Neal Apple M.D. in New Mexico, and attended many Vision Conferences where she gained further insights from various colleagues.

In Esther's early forties the illness and subsequent passing of her niece created eight months of high stress during which she saw her own near vision plummet worryingly. Reading even at arm's length became difficult, and concentration was a challenge for a while. She knew it was time to look closely at her own sight again, and to delve deeper for answers. A six hour palming session helped her regain most of her near vision, and this book is a result of her studies that have kept her free from reading glasses.

Esther is passionate about teaching and loves to let people know that eyesight can improve. She is a member of the North American Association of Vision Educators. She presents conference lectures and workshops and teaches classes and private lessons in the USA and Europe, as well as world-wide through the internet.

Esther currently resides in Ojai, California, where she enjoys life in the sun. ☼
Website: www.visionsofjoy.org